Globalization and Health

An Introduction

Kelley Lee
Senior Lecturer in Global Health Policy
Centre on Global Change and Health
London School of Hygiene & Tropical Medicine,
UK

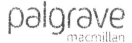
macmillan

© Kelley Lee 2003

Softcover reprint of the hardcover 1st edition 2003 978-0-333-80255-7

First published 2003 by
PALGRAVE MACMILLAN
Houndmills, Basingstoke, Hampshire RG21 6XS and
175 Fifth Avenue, New York, N. Y. 10010
Companies and representatives throughout the world

PALGRAVE MACMILLAN is the global academic imprint of the Palgrave Macmillan division of St. Martin's Press, LLC and of Palgrave Macmillan Ltd. Macmillan® is a registered trademark in the United States, United Kingdom and other countries. Palgrave is a registered trademark in the European Union and other countries.

ISBN 978-1-349-42174-9   ISBN 978-1-4039-4382-8 (eBook)
DOI 10.1057/9781403943828

This book is printed on paper suitable for recycling and made from fully managed and sustained forest sources.

A catalogue record for this book is available from the British Library.

Library of Congress Cataloging-in-Publication Data

Lee, Kelley, 1962-
    Globalization and health : an introduction / Kelley Lee.
        p. cm.
    Includes bibliographical references and index.

        1. Globalization–Health aspects. 2. World health. I. Title.

RA441.L44 2003
362.1–dc21

                                                                    2003042989

10   9   8   7   6   5   4   3   2
12   11   10   09   08   07   06   05

Transferred to digital printing 2005

Global Issues Series

General Editor: **Jim Whitman**

This exciting new series encompasses three principal themes: the interaction of human and natural systems; cooperation and conflict; and the enactment of values. The series as a whole places an emphasis on the examination of complex systems and causal relations in political decision-making; problems of knowledge; authority, control and accountability in issues of scale; and the reconciliation of conflicting values and competing claims. Throughout the series the concentration is on an integration of existing disciplines towards the clarification of political possibility as well as impending crises.

Titles include:

Roy-Carr-Hill and John Lintott
CONSUMPTION, JOBS AND THE ENVIRONMENT
A Fourth Way?

Malcolm Dando
PREVENTING BIOLOGICAL WARFARE
The Failure of American Leadership

Brendan Gleeson and Nicholas Law (*editors*)
GOVERNING FOR THE ENVIRONMENT
Global Problems, Ethics and Democracy

Roger Jeffery and Bhaskar Vira (*editors*)
CONFLICT AND COOPERATION IN PARTICIPATORY NATURAL RESOURCE MANAGEMENT

Ho-Won Jeong (*editor*)
GLOBAL ENVIRONMENTAL POLICIES
Institutions and Procedures
APPROACHES TO PEACEBUILDING

W. Andy Knight
A CHANGING UNITED NATIONS
Multilateral Evolution and the Quest for Global Governance

W. Andy Knight (*editor*)
ADAPTING THE UNITED NATIONS TO A POSTMODERN ERA
Lessons Learned

Kelley Lee
HEALTH IMPACTS OF GLOBALIZATION (*editor*)
Towards Global Governance
GLOBALIZATION AND HEALTH
An Introduction

Nicholas Low and Brendan Gleeson (*editors*)
MAKING URBAN TRANSPORT SUSTAINABLE

Graham S. Pearson
THE UNSCOM SAGA
Chemical and Biological Weapons Non-Proliferation

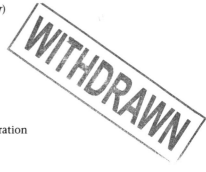

Andrew T. Price-Smith (*editor*)
PLAGUES AND POLITICS
Infectious Disease and International Policy

Michael Pugh (*editor*)
REGENERATION OF WAR-TORN SOCIETIES

Bhaskar Vira and Roger Jeffery (*editors*)
ANALYTICAL ISSUES IN PARTICIPATORY NATURAL RESOURCE MANAGE-
MENT

Simon M. Whitby
BIOLOGICAL WARFARE AGAINST CROPS

Global Issues Series
Series Standing Order ISBN 978-0-333-79483-4
(*outside North America only*)

You can receive future titles in this series as they are published by placing a standing order. Please contact your bookseller or, in case of difficulty, write to us at the address below with your name and address, the title of the series and the ISBN quoted above.

Customer Services Department, Macmillan Distribution Ltd, Houndmills, Basingstoke, Hampshire RG21 6XS, England

To Andrew, Jenny and Alex

Contents

List of Tables, Boxes and Figures

Preface

A defining moment in writing this book came during my visit to the Oldepai* Gorge in northern Tanzania in early 2002 where the oldest remains then known of *Homo erectus* were discovered by Louis and Mary Leakey in 1959. I felt a profound sense of coming full circle standing at the edge of the famous gorge, the 'Cradle of Humankind', where the 'out of Africa' theory seemed to be confirmed. As a Chinese woman of Canadian birth now settled in Europe, my visit to this special place created an appropriate sense of 'globality'. It told me that the globalization story is as old as we are as a species, that much contemporary thinking about the subject fails to contextualize it sufficiently in this important past and, given the constant motion of human beings, it is a continually changing story that remains to be played out in full.

   The subject of this book attempts to provide an introduction to one part of that story, a neglected one so far by globalization scholars, yet a defining one for how human societies have evolved. There are far better historians than myself who have documented the epidemiology of human health and disease over time in relation to the effects on the lives of individuals and communities. There are also far superior scholars of contemporary globalization who have teased apart and put back together the complex strands of the changes currently going on around us. What is missing is the link between the two. Like the Leakeys searching in the red soil for fragments that would help piece together the evolutionary history of hominids, in a far more modest way (and under far more comfortable working conditions), this book seeks to bridge the study of health and globalization in order to shed light on both fields.

   Why the two subjects have so far been such separate endeavours in large part reflects the highly fragmented way that some academic disciplines have developed over the past century, forcing scholars into intellectual pigeonholes that confine their perspective. Individual disciplines can turn in upon themselves, becoming more and more specialized in their hairsplitting of topics familiar to them. In doing so,

---

* This place name is the original spelling as used in Tanzania. The site has come to be known worldwide as the 'Olduvai Gorge' based on a misspelling by Europeans.

they become increasingly obscure to other fields, and fail to share their insights with the uninitiated. The study of globalization and health swims against this tide in recognition that so many of the determinants of health are being impacted upon by processes of global change. Hence the emerging field of global health. But equally important, the trajectory of globalization and its sustainability in the longer term will be directly shaped by a wide range of health-related issues. A better understanding of this symbiotic relationship is the purpose of this introductory text.

Acknowledgements

The writing of such a wide-ranging book has required me to rely on a large number of people to direct me to relevant sources, provide patient explanations of complex and diverse topics, listen to often unformed ideas, and comment on bits of writing. Colleagues and students at the London School of Hygiene & Tropical Medicine have been my biggest source of support, helping to build globalization into a legitimate area of research and teaching in an established international school of public health. My gratitude to Jeff Collin who accepted a ticket to join this growing area of research without realizing how much railway coffee he would have to drink. He has been a highly valued colleague who has stepped in on many occasions to cover all sorts of tasks that a mere mortal would have blanched at. Anna Gilmore has contributed enormously to my thinking around the global dimensions of tobacco control. Karen Bissell has been a key contributor to our team, despite living out of a suitcase, and has been the source of more than one fascinating conversation about the politics of international health. As well as reading earlier drafts, and providing encouragement, Preeti Patel, Sue Lawrence and Barbara Cannito have provided unstinting assistance in obtaining materials for me, including the most obscure papers from the darkest depths of the British Library. Their willingness to find 'something on population growth over time' allowed me to keep the momentum of the writing going. My warm appreciation to my colleagues in the Centre on Global Change and Health, notably Tony McMichael, Paul Wilkinson, Mike Ahern, David Bradley, Ross Mackenzie, Diarmid Campbell-Lendrum, Egbert Sondorp, Carolyn Stephens, Sari Kovats, who have provided ideas and materials on topics touched upon in this book. And my appreciation to Nick Black, Andy Haines, Martin McKee and Dave Leon for continuing to make important space for this work.

A large number of individuals in other institutions have also helped me in the writing of this book. At WHO, I owe thanks to Nick Drager, Robert Beaglehole, Debra Lipson and David Woodward in the Globalization, Trade and Health programme. As well as funding important work that lies behind this book, they have the difficult task of translating scholarly ideas into a form usable by those at the 'coalface' of globalization. My fellow members of the WHO Scientific Resource Group on Globalisation, Trade and Health provided additional comments, notably David Fidler who was the perfect visiting professor, Rene Loewenson and Suwit Wilbulpolprosert. My thanks to Douglas Bettcher and Derek Yach in the Tobacco Free Initiative who have remained a supportive presence, and Guénaël Rodier, Sandy Cocksedge, Maria Santamaria, Mike Ryan and Cathy Roth in Communicable Disease, Surveillance and Response (CSR) for sharing insights into their work. I am also grateful to Johannes Sommerfeld in the Special Programme for Research and Training in Tropical Diseases for involving me in his work.

At The Nuffield Trust, John Wyn Owen, Graham Lister, Sir Maurice Shock and Alan Ingram continue to uniquely bring together the policy and scholarly communities on issues concerning health and globalization. Their creation of the UK Partnership in Global Health (www.ukglobalhealth.org <http://www.ukglobalhealth.org>) has been an important achievement for putting this subject higher on the agendas of national and international policy makers. On a personal note, the Trust's faith in me as a soft-funded researcher looking to build a new area of research has been a clear starting point for this book.

Others who have provided inputs into aspects of this work are Richard Dodgson, Wendy Harcourt, Inge Kaul, Ilona Kickbusch, Ronald Labonte, Tim Lang, Adetokunbo Lucas, John Macmillan, Pim Martens, Craig Murphy, Peter Poore, Alistair Robb, Lance Saker, Jan Aarte Scholte, Anthony So, Eva Wallstram, Morton Warner, Julius Weinberg, Rorden Wilkinson, and Mark Zacher.

For administrative support, I am very grateful to the excellent team of Melanie Batty, Nadja Doyle, Phillip Raponi and Jackie Murphy who provided ongoing and efficient assistance even at the most inopportune moments.

I would like to acknowledge the generous funding of the following organizations which supported some of the research that I have undertaken for this book: US National Institutes of Health Grant No. R01 CA91021-01, Rockefeller Foundation, Nuffield Trust, and World Health Organization.

Finally, I wish to thank my own 'global' family in Canada, the US and UK with whom family ties have become too dependent on emails and post cards. My parents now regularly "close the circle" with visits to our extended family in China. To Anne and Tom Gilmore for providing cover so often and enabling me to travel so extensively. To my husband Andrew with whom I look forward to our next African adventure. And to our two children - I burst with pride watching them learn to left click on a mouse and then wonder what kind of globalized world they will share in decades to come.

Abbreviations

ACHR	Advisory Committee on Health Research
ADD	attention deficit disorder
ADHD	attention deficit hyperactivity disorder
AHEAD	Animal Health/Emerging Animal Disease
AHP	American Home Products
AMR	antimicrobial resistance
ASEAN	Association of South-East Asian Nations
ATC	American Tobacco Company
AZT	Zidovudine
BAT	British American Tobacco
BBC	British Broadcasting Corporation
BMI	body mass index
BMJ	*British Medical Journal*
BSE	bovine spongiform encephalopathy
Bt	*Bacillus thuringiensis*
CAC	Codex Alimentarius Commission
CAP	Common Agricultural Policy (EU)
CARASA	Campaign for Abortion Rights and Against Sterilization Abuse
CDC	US Centers for Disease Control and Prevention (originally Communicable Disease Center)
CEO	Chief Executive Officer
CEPAA	Council on Economic Priorities Accreditation Agency
CHD	coronary heart disease
CME	Commission on Macroeconomics and Health (WHO)
CNTC	China National Tobacco Corporation
COHRED	Council on Health Research for Development
COMESA	Common Market of East and Southern Africa
CSR	corporate social responsibility
CVD	cardiovascular disease
DALE	disability adjusted life expectancy
DALY	disability adjusted life year
DfID	Department for International Development (UK)
DNA	deoxyribonucleic acid
DOE	Department of Energy (US)
DPT	diphtheria, pertussis and tetanus
ECOWAS	Economic Community of West African States

ENHR	Essential National Health Research
ERIDs	emerging and re-emerging infectious diseases
ESAP	economic structural adjustment programme
ETS	environmental tobacco smoke
EU	European Union
FAO	Food and Agriculture Organization
FCTC	Framework Convention on Tobacco Control
FDA	Food and Drug Administration (US)
FDI	foreign direct investment
FMD	foot and mouth disease
GATS	General Agreement on Trade in Services
GATT	General Agreement on Tariffs and Trade
GAVI	Global Alliance for Vaccines and Immunizations
GBD	Global Burden of Disease
GDP	global domestic product
GHG	global health governance
GIS	geographic information systems
GM	genetically modified
GMO	genetically modified organism
GNP	gross national product
GOBI-FFF	growth monitoring, oral rehydration, breastfeeding, immunization, female education, family spacing and food supplements
GP	general practitioner
GPG	global public good
GPPP	global public–private partnership
G7	Group of Seven countries (Canada, France, Germany, Italy, Japan, UK, US)
G8	Group of Eight countries (Canada, France, Germany, Italy, Japan, Russia, UK, US)
GPA	Global Programme on AIDS
GPHIN	Global Public Health Intelligence Network
GSK	GlaxoSmithKline plc
HFA	Health for All
HFEA	Human Fertilization and Embryology Authority (UK)
HGP	Human Genome Project
HIV/AIDS	human immunodeficiency syndrome/acquired immuno-deficiency syndrome
HPI	Human Poverty Index
IARC	International Agency for Research on Cancer
IBFAN	International Baby Food Action Network

ICFTU	International Confederation of Free Trade Unions
ICPD	International Conference on Population and Development
ICTs	information and communication technologies
IDTs	International Development Targets
IDU	intravenous drug user
IFPMA	International Federation of Pharmaceutical Manufacturers Association
IHR	International Health Regulations
ILO	International Labour Organization/Office
ILSI	International Life Sciences Institute
IMF	International Monetary Fund
INB	Intergovernmental Negotiating Body
INFOTAB	International Tobacco Information Centre
IOM	International Organization for Migration
IPCC	Intergovernmental Panel on Climate Change
IPR	intellectual property rights
ISDN	Integrated Services Digital Network
IUCN	International Union for Conservation of Nature and Natural Resources (World Conservation Union)
IVF	*in vitro* fertilization
IWHC	International Women's Health Coalition
JICA	Japanese International Cooperation Agency
LCDC	Laboratory Centre for Disease Control (Canada)
LPI	Living Planet Index
MAI	Multilateral Agreement on Investment
MDRTB	multidrug resistant tuberculosis
MERCOSUR	Market of the South
MHz	megahertz
MMR	mumps, measles and rubella
MRSA	methicillin resistant *Staphylococcus aureas*
MTA	multilateral trade agreement
NAFTA	North American Free Trade Agreement
NCD	noncommunicable disease
NGO	nongovernmental organization
NHS	National Health Service (UK)
NHTSA	National Highway Traffic Safety Administration (US)
NIH	National Institutes of Health (US)
NPA	new public administration
NPM	new public management
NWHN	National Women's Health Network

OAS	Organization of American States
ODA	official development assistance
OECD	Organization for Economic Cooperation and Development
OIHP	Organisation d'Hygiène de Publique
OMNI	Organizing Medical Networked Information
ORT	oral rehydration therapy
OTCs	over the counter drugs
PASB	Pan American Sanitary Bureau
PAHO	Pan American Health Organization
PGD	pre-implantation genetic diagnosis
PHC	primary health care
Plc	public limited company
PMI	Phillip Morris International
PPP	purchasing power parity
ProMED	Programme for Monitoring Emerging Diseases
PSAC	Policy and Strategy Advisory Committee
R&D	research and development
RBF	regular budget funds
SAP	structural adjustment programme
SARS	Sudden Acute Respiratory Syndrome
SCF	Save the Children Fund
SE	*Salmonella serotype Enteritidis*
SIDA	Swedish International Development Cooperation Agency
SPS	Agreement on Sanitary and Phytosanitary Standards
STD	sexually transmitted disease
TNCs	transnational corporations
TRIPS	Agreement on Trade-Related Intellectual Property Rights
TTCs	transnational tobacco companies
TWG	Transitional Working Group
UK	United Kingdom
UN	United Nations
UNAIDS	United Nations Joint Programme on HIV/AIDS
UNCTAD	United Nations Conference on Trade and Development
UNDP	United Nations Development Programme
UNESCO	United Nations Educational, Social and Cultural Organization
UNFPA	United Nations Population Fund
UNHCR	United Nations High Commissioner for Refugees
UNICEF	United Nations Children's Fund
UNRRA	United Nations Relief and Rehabilitation Administration

US	United States
USAID	United States Agency for International Development
USDA	United States Department of Agriculture
vCJD	variant Creutzfeldt-Jakob disease
VISA	Vancomycin Intermediate-Resistant *Staphylococcus aureas*
WBCSD	World Business Council on Sustainable Development
WDR	World Development Report
WHA	World Health Assembly
WHO	World Health Organization
WIPO	World Intellectual Property Organization
WSMI	World Self-Medication Industry
WTO	World Tourism Organization
WTO	World Trade Organization
WWF	Worldwide Fund for Nature

1
An Introduction to Global Health

1.1 Introduction

The profusion of scholarly and policy debates surrounding globalization over the past decade or so has been both abundant and wide-ranging in subject matter, approach and conclusions. From a starting point of documenting the trend towards increasing interdependence among countries, the field has grown into a major endeavour whose outputs threaten to overwhelm even the keenest reader. The aim of this book is not simply to add to this relentlessly growing mountain of literature, much of which remains highly contested. Rather, its purpose is to address a surprising gap, namely the links between globalization and human health, a subject that so far occupies a relatively minor corner in broader debates. Indeed, much emphasis continues to be placed on the economic and technological aspects of globalization. There is thus a surfeit of treatises on the detailed machinations of the so-called emerging global economy, the various forces driving its seemingly inexorable spread, and the many ways it could best be managed by various levels of governance. These debates undoubtedly remain highly central to understanding the key features of continuity and change in the emerging world order.

Posing clear challenges to the indiscriminate impacts of current forms of economic globalization is a diverse collection of voices. Initially a rather dispersed collection of issues, by the late 1990s these concerns had mobilized into a significant force, embracing a broad swathe of the political spectrum. The unifying theme is a belief that the social and environmental consequences of globalization are being given insufficient consideration amid the onward march towards a global economy. The most visible expression of these concerns has been the mass 'anti-globalization' protests since the late 1990s, organized to coincide with high-level meetings of world leaders. Equally important, however, has been the formation of advocacy groups, research centres, policy forums and discussion websites devoted to generating and disseminating information, as well as building links with like-minded groups. The rapid proliferation of such initiatives, and their willingness to intervene in a variety of scholarly and policy debates, reflect substantial levels of concern about the current nature and direction of economic globalization. Even the most hardened advocates of unfettered globalization acknowledge that there is a need, at the very least, to consider how globalization impacts upon aspects of human life beyond the marketplace.

In recent years, it is into this highly contested arena that questions about the positive and negative impacts of globalization on human health have arisen. Health-related issues cut across a wide range of debates about globalization:

- the extent to which the erosion of national sovereignty will affect a state's capacity to set national health policy and raise sufficient resources for health care;
- the degree to which the protection of public health is provided for in multilateral trade agreements under the World Trade Organization (WTO);
- the effect of global marketing practices by large transnational corporations (TNCs);
- the migration of industrial waste and hazards across countries and regions;
- the influence on health and safety standards as a result of the worldwide mobility of capital and investment;
- the link between widening socioeconomic inequities within and across countries, and their subsequent effects on health status for adversely affected population groups;
- the relationship between global climate change, distribution of vectors of disease and epidemiological trends;
- the changing patterns of health and disease from intensified population mobility and new patterns of human settlement;
- the potential for global information and communication technologies to enhance public health information, disease surveillance and the provision of health care services;
- the health threat posed by the global proliferation of the arms trade, biological weapons, terrorist activities, illicit drug trafficking, tobacco smuggling and other criminal activities;

- the global spread of values, beliefs and practices that may have positive or negative effects on health;
- the mobilization of greater resources for global health initiatives;
- and the changing balance of power among key public and private sector actors in health.

All of these issues and more have been raised as part of the emerging 'global health agenda'. It is loud and clear, therefore, that the health community has added its voice to the chorus of concerned individuals and groups worldwide who want to see more socially conscious and humane forms of globalization.

In order to give optimal weight to concerns about human health as a result of globalization, it is important to distinguish between those issues that have genuinely arisen as a consequence of global change and those that the health community has faced *a priori*. The health community is as guilty as other fields in its overuse and misuse of the term 'global', including the tendency to repackage old woes to give them a new lease of life. Pushed to the extreme by a kind of Gaia theory[1] gone berserk, everything is poured into the globalization pot that, in turn, becomes demonized as responsible for a vast range of social and environmental ills. While this may indeed be true, the capacity to demonstrate this in a politically convincing way is diluted by imprecision of definition, lack of conceptual clarity and insufficient empirical evidence. There is a need, in short, to demonstrate where globalization gives a particular twist to existing health issues and where it poses new challenges altogether. Clear conceptualization of the links between globalization and human health includes a coherent framework for locating these links within the broader debates about globalization, and that offers insights into the particular issues that arise in relation to health.

It is this task that underlies the purpose of this book. In this introductory chapter, a brief discussion of the meaning of globalization and its defining characteristics is followed by a conceptual framework for understanding the links between globalization and health. A discussion of the distinction between international and global health is then presented, supporting the need to expand current thinking about both globalization and health. This introduction then sets the scene for more in-depth analysis in the following chapters, accompanied by empirical examples throughout to illustrate the diversity of these links, and the imperative need to address them more actively through research and policy.

1.2   What is globalization?

In wading into the globalization debate, almost immediately it is necessary to draw a line in the sand to show where we stand on a range of issues if we are to avoid falling victim to intellectual vagueness and imprecision. Invariably, this is a tricky challenge because one immediately confronts the fact that globalization is 'amongst the most abused and misused terms in popular usage' (Jones 1995: 3). First, there is no one agreed definition of globalization because the concept is inseparable from different value-based views of the way the world works and ought to work. The descriptive is bound inextricably with the prescriptive and normative. Second, the term 'global' is often used interchangeably with such terms as international and world, resulting in further confusion of meaning. Third, the abundant literature available comes from many disciplines, with each focusing on selected aspects of globalization that are seen to be of definitive importance – economists emphasize flows of capital, goods and services; political scientists are concerned with emerging power structures and balances; environmentalists give attention to impacts on ecological systems; management consultants explore how corporations can expand and operate globally. In certain fields, such as economics, international relations/politics, development studies, cultural studies, business and management, and sociology, the initiated are blessed with some degree of theoretical and empirical writing. For those in the health field, as relative latecomers to the globalization field of battle, the apparently sensible strategy of borrowing from intellectual foundations laid in other subject areas is not unproblematic either if done uncritically. Hence, the issue of definition is heavily contingent on distinguishing among different schools of thought, values, political ideologies, levels of analyses, epistemologies and other provisos.

Mercifully, a number of excellent works have been published in recent years that help us along the path towards a clearer synthesis of the key issues at hand. Rather than delving into a long and laboured discussion here of the intricacies of globalization, a feat already achieved to such a high standard elsewhere, this book draws on these selected works to map out the major points of contention. This is done to arrive at a working definition of globalization, and to build the conceptual framework presented below for understanding and responding to the links between globalization and health.

The first point of contention, and perhaps the most fundamental, is whether globalization is happening or not. There is no shortage of detractors who argue either that nothing is happening at all, or that something is happening but it is not qualitatively new. The main evidence cited for this focuses on economic globalization, describable as 'a process of rapid economic integration driven by the liberalisation of trade, investment and capital flows, as well as by rapid technological change and the "Information Revolution"' (Oxfam 2000: 10). Challenging the stronger versions of economic globalization, as advocated by such writers as Ohmae (1995), Hirst and Thompson (1995) argue that the 'present highly internationalised economy is not unprecedented', and that comparably high levels of international trade can be found from the second half of the nineteenth century. They also point to the concentration of trade, investment and financial flows in the triad of Europe, Japan and North America, and the rarity of genuine transnational corporations (TNCs) as evidence of the limited 'global' nature of the world economy.

Such scepticism about the newness of globalization has been taken to task by a number of writers for using a narrow and idealized definition of globalization, hence failing to acknowledge important developments in the world economy. Eschewing 'all or nothing' approaches to globalization, these writers recognize the continuity of the international (states-based) economy, and the uneven pace of change that is occurring. Dicken (1998), for example, argues that we are witnessing the emergence of a new geo-economy with a qualitatively different structure, one that encompasses processes of both internationalization and globalization. *Internationalization* processes 'involve the simple extension of economic activities across national boundaries'. He writes that this is essentially a quantitative change that is leading to more intensive and extensive geographical patterns of economic activity. In contrast, *globalization* processes 'involve not merely the geographical extension of economic activity across national boundaries but also – and more importantly – the *functional integration* [original italics] of such internationally dispersed activities'. This 'global shift' is a qualitative change whereby the world economy is 'being transformed into a highly complex, kaleidoscope structure involving the fragmentation of many production processes and their geographical relocation on a global scale in ways which slice through national boundaries'. Hence, a transition of some kind is believed to be taking place, from industrialization to modernization or even 'post' or 'late' modernization, a phase sometimes called the post-industrial or post-Fordist economy. The defining features of this emerging order are broadly recognized in terms of the following characteristics:

- a shift from heavy industry and manufacturing to a greater proportion of services provision;
- an increase in economic activities concerned with the generation, processing and dissemination of information;
- a deeper degree of economic integration, from arm's length trade in goods and services between independent firms and international movements of portfolio capital, to close linkages in the production of goods and services across national boundaries;
- a trend in production and consumption towards larger economies of scale from the subnational and national to regional and global scale; and
- a higher degree of mobility of capital, goods and services, and to a more limited degree selected sections of the labour market.

Importantly, responses to sceptics about globalization also hold that the processes of change at work go far beyond the economic sphere, to involve broader social and environmental processes. While economic change may arguably be leading and, indeed even driving, processes of globalization, the economic is more frequently seen as part of a wide-ranging set of complex changes to human societies as a whole. Pieterse (1995) describes globalization as 'a multi-dimensional process which, like all significant social processes, unfolds in multiple realms of existence simultaneously ... there are many modes of globalization as there are globalizing agents and dynamics or impulses'. Similarly, Giddens (1990) refers to 'the intensification of worldwide social relations which link distant localities in such a way that local happenings are shaped by events occurring many miles away and vice versa.' We might thus think of globalization in the plural – economic globalization, political globalization, environmental globalization, sociocultural globalization and so on – processes that are multiple yet intimately interrelated. Such an approach fits well with understanding the links between globalization and health. While economic structures and forces play a key role in determining health outcomes, their role cannot be understood apart from the social context as a whole.

A second point of debate revolves around causative explanations of how globalization occurs. It is often implied that globalization has a rational momentum of its own, driven by some assumed logic of, for example, the 'invisible hand' of the free market or 'natural evolution'

of human societies. This, in turn, leads to assumptions about globalization as apolitical or value-neutral, guided by an inherent rationalism
rather than vested interests, and on balance a progressive force. It is
these types of arguments that lie behind frequent claims that we
cannot stop globalization but rather we must somehow adapt to its
inexorable spread. Faced with this unstoppable force, opposition to
globalization, regulation or redirection of its drivers, or mitigation of
some of its effects, is seen as misguided at best, and interfering in
progress at worst.

It is a starting point of this book, however, that a clear distinction
should be made between the terms global change and globalization.
Global change can be described as change whose origins or impacts are
transborder (they transcend politically defined state boundaries or
borders) with some even rendering territorial geography obsolete.
Many forms of environmental change, for example, are global because
their causes (such as the creation of carbon dioxide) do not respect
national borders, nor do their consequences (such as ozone depletion).
It is further useful to differentiate between two causes of global change.
The first are *naturally-induced* global changes, those changes that have
causal origins in nature. The world's climate, for instance, has been
changing for millions of years, with the last great cooling occurring
around 250 million years ago at the end of the Permian era when the
continents coalesced into Pangaea. One result was the extinction of
nine-tenths of existing life forms, giving way to the evolution of reptiles and dinosaurs during the Triassic and Jurassic periods (McMichael
2001). All sorts of global changes have occurred, and continue to
occur, as a result of natural processes. *Human-induced* (anthropogenic)
global change are those that are caused by human behaviour and
actions. The migration of *Homo erectus* beginning about one million
years ago, and later *Homo sapiens*, from Africa to other continents
invariably brought with it impacts on the natural environment as communities formed, settlements were established and natural resources
used. More recently, the establishment of megacities, burning of fossil
fuels and industrialization of agriculture have all had global impacts.

It is human-induced global change that this book refers to as *globalization*. While there are clear impacts on the natural world of many
forms of globalization, it is human activity individually and collectively that ultimately drives globalization. The particular form that it
takes, how its effects are assessed and responded to, and even how it is
understood therefore lie within the power of people to direct, guide
and control it. Such power is undoubtedly unequally distributed, and

one of the great challenges remains the enfranchisement of a wider constituency to contribute to its definition. There is thus a need to demystify globalization, to challenge its political origins and trajectories, and to assert direction and control over its parameters and impacts. As individuals, we are indeed subject to the forces of change around us but, collectively, we are also responsible for the sum of decisions we take to define the nature of globalization.

Third, the argument that globalization, as a new phenomenon, has been overstated hinges on the perceived timescale involved. Many writers hold that globalization is a relatively recent phenomenon, defined foremost by the expansion of the world economy since the late twentieth century (Rugman and Gestrin 1997). Increasingly, however, these recent changes are recognized as part of a longer historical process. Robertson (1992), for example, argues that globalization comprises several historical forms or stages dating from around 1500, with each stage characterized by particular features of modern society and a nascent global system. Giddens (1990) defines globalization in terms of four dimensions – world-military order, national-state system, world capitalist economy, and international division of labour. These 'institutions of modernity' similarly date from the fourteenth century. In his discussion of globalization in history, Scholte (2000) also traces some aspects of the spread of supraterritoriality back several centuries.

Importantly, all these authors distinguish between the historical origins of globalization, and developments of more recent decades in the form of an acceleration of globalization. The period from about the late 1960s is widely identified as a turning point in the historical unfolding of globalization processes, marked by such diverse events as the landing on the moon, increased use of transoceanic cables, satellite communications and other information technologies, spread of transborder production and consumption patterns, and the expansion of global organizations. Scholte (2000: 74) describes this period as 'full-scale globalization' and Robertson (1992: 59) as 'the uncertainty phase'. The main point here is that it is critical to understand the historical particularities of the global changes taking place, and to locate them within an appropriate timescale. The definition of globalization and conceptual framework developed in this book, in relation to health impacts, is based on a view of globalization as a set of processes occurring over many centuries, with particular features defining its precise nature at different points in history. This historical perspective on the links between globalization and health is presented in detail in Chapter 2.

A fourth, and perhaps the most divisive, point of contention about globalization is the nature of the consequences of globalization for selected individuals and population groups. Globalization has been both applauded and blamed for all sorts of good and ill, in many cases without sufficient empirical evidence. Globalization is indeed an apparent bundle of contradiction, an embodiment of the 'Push me, Pull you' creature of Dr Doolittle fame. Its attributed features include:

- a generator of greater wealth or creator of widening socioeconomic inequalities;
- a source of widespread social integration across countries or disintegration among fragmenting social groupings and structures;
- a creator of shared identities or a force of division and alienation;
- a process leading to a 'borderless world' and 'end of geography' or reinforcer of nationalism and regionalism;
- an enabler of democracy and equity, or a major contributor to widening gaps between 'haves' and 'have nots'; and
- a facilitator of greater cooperation or competition among individuals and groups.

To a large extent, the variability in views about globalization can be ascribed to the existence of diverse theoretical, disciplinary and ideological identities described above. In broad brushstrokes, liberal-based theories (including neoliberalism and rational choice theory) have been the most positive advocates of globalization. Globalization is hailed as the progress of market capitalism triumphing on a worldwide scale, a logical continuation of the mercantilism of the eighteenth century, European colonization, industrialization of Europe, North America and gradually other parts of the world. The essence of this perspective lies in the freedom of the individual, unfettered by overly cumbersome social restrictions, in their pursuit of happiness through, *inter alia*, the accumulation of material wealth. By allowing individuals and groups to express this entrepreneurial energy, it is assumed that this wealth eventually 'trickles down' to benefit society as a whole. Overall, this is held to be an essentially rational and progressive process that, if allowed to run its course, increases the efficiency and productivity of economies.

Globalization is seen as an extension of liberal economic theory to a larger scale to encompass economic activity across all countries. Liberalism is believed to embody universal principles that, through competitive market forces and the pursuit of greater economies of scale, leads subnationally and nationally based economic entities to expand outwards beyond the state. Hence, globalization means that countries of the so-called developing world and former socialist bloc are converging, with western industrialized countries, towards a single global economic system. This emerging global economy, with flows of capital, labour, and goods and services across national borders with minimal interference, is eventually expected to create material benefits for all (Ohmae 1990). Any bumps along the way are due to continued interference with free markets through excess regulation of markets, or simply a failure to allow a sufficiently long timeframe for the processes to have their intended effect. This essentially Panglossian view of the drivers of globalization, as a liberal utopia, has been most widely associated with the so-called Washington Consensus.[2]

Responses to this vision of globalization have focused on sharply refuting its underlying assumptions, and warning of its destabilizing, destructive and ultimately unsustainable impacts. Of particular note is what Falk (1999: 1–3) describes as the change in relative strength 'between global capital and governments operating at the level of the sovereign state', resulting in the undermining of 'the capacity of the state to contribute to human well-being'. He refers to now-familiar neoliberal policy prescriptions, led by privatization, deregulation and the rolling back of the welfare state, as 'predatory globalization' because of its cumulatively adverse effects on human well-being, notably through the erosion of the social contract between the state and society that was forged during the previous century. Thus, a growing body of empirical work is drawing attention to the costs of current forms of globalization that go beyond the economic. These social, environmental and political costs are at present insufficiently addressed, resulting in an exacerbation of divisions between the 'haves' and 'have nots' of the world (Amin 1997). This is manifest, for instance, in the decline of the welfare state, weakened labour standards, increased employment insecurity and greater social exclusion (Kennedy 1996; Wilding 1997). Concerns over the intended and unintended consequences of neoliberal-defined globalization have led to predictions that it will eventually succumb to its own internal contradictions (Cox 1995).

What is evident from these polarized perspectives and somewhat contradictory evidence about globalization is that they reflect the highly varied impacts being created for different individuals and population groups. There are undoubtedly both positive and negative impacts of globalization, simultaneously bringing costs and benefits in varying proportions to different people. In this respect, globalization can be distinguished from the term *interdependence* which has been used to suggest mutual dependence (and hence mutual costs and benefits). Globalization generates relationships of *dependence*, with inequitable sharing of costs and benefits, as well as reinforces existing inequalities. Critical theorists, in particular, are concerned with the losers of 'uneven globalization' – those who experience increased economic insecurity, political alienation and social exclusion. The winners from globalization, in contrast, are advantaged by greater resources, mobility and opportunities to enjoy the fruits of change. Not surprisingly, whether one feels that globalization is having positive or negative consequences depends on the particular vision of globalization one holds, as well as one's place within this emerging pecking order. One of the key challenges for research and policy making, therefore, is to better understand how globalization is impacting on different individuals and groups, what those specific impacts are, and how they could be mediated.

Between the optimism of neoliberal-based perspectives, with the focus on the 'winners' of globalization, and more critical perspectives focusing on the 'losers', many scholars and policy makers are struggling to come to terms with the implications of globalization for particular areas of human activity. Fundamental divisions remain over whether these impacts are temporary blips on a generally upward trajectory towards greater wealth, health and democracy for all, or whether the current system is inherently flawed and ultimately unsustainable. Policy prescriptions thus veer between tinkering with globalizing forces and fundamental restructuring. The World Bank (2000), for example, accepts that 'the extent to which different countries participate in [economic] globalization is far from uniform'. The problem is perceived here as too little, rather than too much, integration into this emerging order: 'For many of the poorest least-developed countries the problem is not that they are being impoverished by globalization, but that they are in danger of being largely excluded from it.' In contrast, so-called anti-globalization protesters have mobilized around their shared exclusion from the globally powerful alliances being formed among big businesses and big governments, attacking WTO negotiations and McDonald restaurants as symbols of this emerging order. A more moderate response, and one that accepts the need for a range of responses to the diverse impacts of globalization, would seek 'to work toward their [capital-driven forces] containment and partial transformation by reference to widely shared world order values' (Falk 1999: 3).

Importantly, this brief review shows that, despite being a highly contested and diversely interpreted phenomenon, distinctive characteristics of globalization can be usefully identified. This book seeks to steer a steady course through this Charybdis of debate, seeking to find ways of better understanding how the health consequences of globalization fit into this complex picture. It rejects the polarized nature that is increasingly characterizing the health debate on globalization (Lee 2001a), in favour of clearer definition, description, measurement and prescription. To summarize the points of debate so far, therefore, and to move towards a working definition for this book, it is recognized that:

- globalization is a qualitatively distinct phenomenon whose particular features are confused by its conflation with terms such as liberalization, colonization, westernization and internationalization;
- globalization is a human-induced and driven set of processes, and is not caused by some inherent logic or rationalism towards a necessarily progressive end;
- globalization is an historical and nonlinear process that has been unfolding over centuries, rather than decades, with developments since the mid to late twentieth century suggesting we are currently within a particularly intense phase of globalization; and
- globalization is a complex and uneven process that is leading to varying, sometimes contradictory, consequences for different individuals and population groups, and resulting in both winners and losers, risks and opportunities.

From these starting points, a working definition of globalization for the purposes of this book is *a set of processes that are changing the nature of human interaction by intensifying interactions across certain boundaries that have hitherto served to separate individuals and population groups.* These spatial, temporal and cognitive boundaries, described in detail below, have become increasingly eroded, resulting in new forms of social organization and interaction across these boundaries. The resulting impacts are evident across many spheres of human society – economic, political, cultural, technological and so on. This definition suggests that the most immediate task at hand is to describe in greater detail the defining features of globalization and to understand its particular implications for human health. For this purpose, we now turn to the development of a conceptual framework for analyzing globalization and health.

1.3 Globalization and health: a conceptual framework

Given the contested nature of so many aspects of globalization, the task of comprehending its implications, let alone responding to the changes being brought about, is a daunting task. As Weick (1999: 39) describes, 'Global issues that involve organizing on a massive scale have been described as contested, nonlinear metaproblems with long lead times, unintended side effects, unclear cause–effect structures, and consequences that are often irreversible.' Despite the challenges, there has been growing impetus since the mid 1990s to address the health impacts of globalization for three reasons.

The first arises from widespread concerns over the social impacts of globalization, spurred by accumulating evidence that all is far from well with the emerging world around us. Undoubtedly, unprecedented progress in health status was achieved over the twentieth century. Life expectancy at birth has increased faster worldwide in the recent past than it did in the preceding 4000 years. Between 1980 and 1998, average life expectancy at birth increased from 61 to 67 years, or an average of four months each year since 1970. The most dramatic gains have occurred in low- and middle-income countries as a result of increased access to nutritious foods,[3] primary health care and education. Child death rates have also halved since 1965, with infant mortality rates falling from 80 to 54 per 1000 live births between 1980 and 1998 (World Bank 1998). These remarkable improvements in the quality of nutrition, housing, water and sanitation, and other basic human needs have enabled human populations to expand at unprecedented rates. After many thousands of years, the world's population reached one billion in 1825. Within one hundred years, this figure doubled to two billion, half a century later (1925–76) to four billion (Thomas 1979), and 25 years later (2001) to six billion people (UNFPA 2002).

However, aggregate data conceal substantial variations within and across countries. Life expectancy at birth varies from 81 years in Japan to 41 years in Rwanda. Infant mortality differences between OECD countries and the developing world declined in absolute terms (from 86 in 1970 to 53 in 1999) but rose in relative terms from five to ten times as high. In 11 countries, including North Korea, Zimbabwe and Kenya, infant mortality has increased. In sub-Saharan Africa, child mortality rates increased between 1990 and 1999 from 155 to 161 per 1000 live births (World Bank 2001). There are also marked differences by gender, with women living on average seven to eight years longer in high-income countries, but female babies and children facing a greater risk of mortality under five than male children in some cultural settings (WHO 2000d). Similar differentials can be observed for race, socioeconomic class, and level of education.

There remains substantial debate about the precise impacts of globalization on specific population groups. Data on economic growth and its relationship to standard of living remain difficult to interpret for subnational and transnational populations because of the form of available data and how they are interpreted. A review of current evidence by Wade (2001), for example, suggests that global inequality has worsened rapidly in recent decades amid the acceleration of globalization. These data use measures such as purchasing power parity (PPP) and the Gini coefficient[4] to calculate world income distribution, and is concerned with income distribution among the world's population regardless of country or region. Milanovic (2000) and Dikhanov and Ward (2001) find that the rate of increase of inequality was faster between 1988 and 1993 than during the 1980s, with the Gini coefficient increasing from 62.5 to 66.0. Measures of socioeconomic inequality over time show that inequality has been growing within many countries since the early 1980s. Argentina, Chile, Colombia, Costa Rica, Uruguay and China experienced increased income inequality alongside trade liberalization during the past three decades. Other measures of world income distribution show similar trends. In 1960 average per capita gross domestic product (GDP) in the richest twenty countries was fifteen times that of the poorest twenty countries. Three decades later this gap had increased to thirty times, a result of relatively faster economic growth in richer countries (World Bank 2000). UNDP (1999:2) reports a similar widening of the income gap between the one-fifth of the world's population living in the wealthiest countries and the one-fifth living in the poorest countries, rising from 30:1 in 1960 to 74:1 in 1997. More than eighty countries, largely in Africa and eastern and central Europe, have experienced declining per capita incomes since 1990. Put succinctly, 10 per cent of the world's population receives 70 per cent of its total income and produces 70 per cent of its goods and services (Wolf 2001).

Voices for forms of globalization based on values of social justice come from many sources (Box 1.1). Domestically, politicians in many higher-income countries have sought a middle ground or 'third way' between the individualist policies of free market capitalism that dominated the 1980s, and the more communitarian values of social democracy (Giddens 1998). As George (1999) writes: 'Business and the market have their place, but this place cannot occupy the entire sphere of human existence.' Extended to the global level, where the end of the Cold War left somewhat of a development policy vacuum, global initiatives to tackle poverty, cancel foreign debt and build social infrastructures have gained momentum. As Wade (2001: 97) writes,

> Growing inequality is analogous to global warming. Its effects are diffuse and long-term, and there is always something more pressing to deal with. The question is how much more unequal world income distribution can become before the resulting political instabilities and flows of migrants reach the point of directly harming the well-being of the citizens of the rich world and the stability of their states.

In the early twenty-first century, therefore, we are searching for how best to manage the forces of globalization, to shape it so that benefits accrue to the greatest number of people, and that they do so in an environmentally sustainable and socially just manner. Even among the most hardened globalists, there is sufficient disquiet to elicit a flurry of policy debate about the pros and cons of globalization for human welfare (World Bank 2000).

The protection and promotion of health has been recognized since the mid 1990s as a core element of such efforts to promote socially and environmentally responsible forms of globalization, including the need to identify and address 'health gaps' within and between countries. As described above, there is growing evidence of the links between globalization and income inequality. Putting this evidence together with well-established links between inequality and health status (Wilkinson 1996) raises clear concerns about the adverse impacts of globalization on the health status of disadvantaged populations. Just as the globalizing world of today is one marred by striking inequalities and unevenness in the sharing of opportunities and risks, so too is this reflected in the health sector. This is illustrated by the following statistics:

- in South Africa, infant mortality is five times higher among blacks than whites, while in certain populations in Russia, China and Chile, gaps in life expectancy are widening over time with evidence of a net deterioration in health (Rockefeller Foundation 2001);
- more than 90 per cent of HIV infections are in the developing world (UK DfID 2000);

Box 1.1 Diverse expressions of concern over the social and environmental consequences of globalization

'Globalisation creates unprecedented new opportunities and risks. If the poorest countries can be drawn into the global economy and get increasing access to modern knowledge and technology, it could lead to a rapid reduction in global poverty – as well as bringing new trade and investment opportunities for all. But if this is not done, the poorest countries will become more marginalised, and suffering and division will grow. And we will all be affected by the consequences.'

UK Prime Minister Tony Blair, as quoted in UK 2000

'Over the last century the forces of globalization have been among those that have contributed to a huge improvement in human welfare, including raising countless millions out of poverty. Going forward, these forces have the potential to continue bringing great benefits to the poor, but how strongly they do so will also continue to depend crucially on factors such as the quality of overall macroeconomic policies, the workings of institutions, both formal and informal, the existing structure of assets, and the available resources, among many others.'

World Bank, *Assessing Globalization*, April 2000

'the view that globalisation is inherently bad for the poor is wrong, what matters is that globalisation is managed in a way that extends opportunities for poor people by overcoming the disadvantages linked to their poverty'

Oxfam, *Globalization*, May 2000

'the social impact of globalization as it is currently conceived and managed is much wider ... The need is now for a socially responsible globalization (globalization with a human face) which combines global trade and investment with global (and regional) social redistribution, global (and regional) social regulation, and global (and regional) social empowerment of citizens everywhere.'

Bob Deacon, 'Global Social Policy', in Deacon et al. 1997

'if globalization is properly interpreted and practised it can result in a more equitable world order where wealth is more evenly distributed between the rich and the poor. Badly interpreted it can destroy the poor especially and by extension stifle the growth of the rich.'

Malaysian Prime Minister Mahathir Bin Mohamed, 2000

'The central challenge we face today is to ensure that globalization becomes a positive force for all the world's people, instead of leaving billions of them behind in squalor. Inclusive globalization must be built on the great enabling force of the market, but market forces alone will not achieve it. It requires a broader effort to create a shared future, based upon our common humanity in all its diversity.'

UN Secretary General Kofi Annan, *Report to the Millennium Assembly*, 2000

- in the US the incidence of HIV/AIDS among women is increasing more rapidly than among men, rising threefold in 1985–94, 77 per cent of cases among black and Hispanic women (Farmer 1999:265);
- the poorest 20 per cent of the world's population have a fourteenfold higher risk of death in childhood than the richest 20 per cent;
- more people than at any other time in history are dying from TB (up to three million annually), with about 95 per cent of the 8 million cases reported each year in the developing world (Fanning 1998);
- tobacco-related diseases will kill 10 million people annually by 2030 of which 70 per cent will occur in the developing world (Yach and Bettcher 2000);
- more than 880 million people lack access to health services, and 2.6 billion lack access to basic sanitation (UNDP 1999);
- less than 10 per cent of total global spending (1992 estimate of US$56 billion) on health research is devoted to 90 per cent of the world's health problems (Global Forum for Health Research 2000); and
- nearly 30 per cent of deaths in the developing world are from infectious diseases yet they receive only 1.5 per cent of foreign aid (WHO 1999).

A second impetus behind increased attention to the links between globalization and health has come from the sometimes alarmist fears that ill-health, largely although not exclusively in the form of infectious diseases, can spread from poorer to richer countries as a result of global change. Since the mid 1990s, the end of the Cold War has encouraged a shift in attention from traditional (largely military) national security concerns towards 'new' security threats such as environmental degradation, population growth and migration, illicit criminal activity, terrorism and health risks. The latter has provoked public concern with the return of plague and pestilence, fuelled by a substantial popular literature preoccupied with the nastiest features of such diseases as Ebola, HIV/AIDS and drug-resistant forms of tuberculosis (Preston 1994; Karlen 1995; Peters and Olshaker 1997; Ryan 1996). Death and disease have become bestsellers among the relatively affluent in high-income countries who had assumed that infectious diseases were a thing of the past or at least could be confined to the developing world. Perhaps the best known of these works is Laurie Garrett's *The Coming Plague* (1994). As well as capturing growing public worry, the book's review of emerging and re-emerging diseases directly

captures the concern among policy makers about the health consequences of globalization. In the preface to *The Coming Plague*, the late
Jonathan Mann, former head of the WHO Global Programme on AIDS,
wrote,

> The world has rapidly become much more vulnerable to the erup-
> tion and, most critically, to the widespread and even global spread
> of both new and old infectious diseases. This new and heightened
> vulnerability is not mysterious. The dramatic increases in worldwide
> movement of people, goods, and ideas is the driving force behind
> the globalization of disease ... The lesson is that a health problem in
> any part of the world can rapidly become a health threat to many or
> all.

This wedding of the emerging global health agenda with realist-based
notions of national security has resulted in the elevation of some
health issues to 'high' politics.[5] Since the late 1980s global health
issues have received increasing attention within high-level policy
circles, particularly in the United States. In 1999 a special assistant was
appointed to the National Security Advisor for international health
affairs, and the United States National Security Strategy for the twenty-
first century accords global health a place alongside arms control and
major theatre warfare (White House 1999). This was followed by a
report of the US National Intelligence Council (2000) which concluded
that 'New and re-emerging infectious diseases will pose a rising global
health threat and will complicate US and global security over the next
20 years ... These diseases will endanger US citizens at home and
abroad, threaten US armed forces deployed overseas, and exacerbate
social and political instability in key countries and regions in which
the United States has significant interests'. Reports by the Institutes of
Medicine (1997) and Council on Foreign Relations and Milbank
Memorial Fund (Kassalow 2001), and the Center for Domestic and
International Health Security initiative by the influential think tank
RAND (2002), set out the same message – health issues are part of the
new security agenda. These concerns were underscored further by the
aftermath of the terrorist bombing of the World Trade Center in
September 2001 when fears of biological and chemical weapons
created new public alarm (PAHO 2001). Diseases have become a
weapon of so-called 'asymmetric warfare' (Nye 2002).
    Internationally, the theme of global health is being carried forth
within a number of prominent forums for the first time (Box 1.2). In

January 2000 the UN Security Council addressed a health and development issue for the first time by highlighting the threat to peace and
security of the HIV/AIDS pandemic. This was followed in July 2000
with the adoption of the first health-related UN Security Council resolution (Resolution 1308) emphasizing the need to combat the spread of
the virus during peacekeeping operations. In June 2001, the UN
General Assembly held a Special Session on HIV/AIDS because the
disease had emerged as a global threat to both human and national
security. The Declaration of Commitment adopted at the meeting contained strategies for dealing with HIV/AIDS in conflict and disaster-
affected regions, and among uniformed personnel (UNAIDS 2001).
Similarly, health has begun to play an increasingly prominent role on
the agendas of Group of Seven (G7) and Group of Eight (G8) summits
beginning in June 2000. Amid tension over trade and other issues of
contention, and vocal demonstrations by anti-globalization protesters,
health cooperation has been a means of building and maintaining
goodwill. Hence, the creation of the Global Fund to Fight HIV/AIDS,
Tuberculosis and Malaria at the G8 Summit in Genoa in June 2001 was
accompanied by commitments by the wealthiest countries to halve the
infectious disease burden by 50 per cent by 2010. Similar discussions
have been held at the World Economic Forum, attended by government leaders, corporate executives and other prominent individuals,
held annually in Davos, Switzerland. All of these initiatives have been
related to what the Director-General of the World Health Organization
(WHO) Gro Harlem Brundtland (2000a) describes as 'health security'.

A third impetus behind growing attention to global health comes
from within the health community itself, prompted by a certain degree
of disquiet at the effectiveness by which it is coping with the changing
world around it. In part, this has arisen from efforts to reform international health cooperation, largely but not primarily focused on the role
of WHO. Since the early 1990s, there has been substantial analysis of
the reform of health-related international organizations amid shifting
epidemiological trends, the emergence of new actors, paradigmatic
shifts in ideology and values, and pressures on resources (Godlee 1994;
Lee et al. 1996; Vaughan et al. 1995; Lucas et al. 1997). While a wide
range of reform issues were raised by these initiatives (Lee 1998c), a
change in WHO leadership in the late 1990s was accompanied by new
hope that health cooperation would be reinvigorated around 'global
health' (Williams 1998). Kickbusch (1997), for example, argues for a
'new public health' which *inter alia* addresses the challenges of globalization through involvement of private sector players, the health care

---

Box 1.2   Global health on the agenda of high-level policy forums

May 1996	G7 Environment Ministers' Meeting includes protection of public health on the agenda for the first time.
January 2000	UN Security Council highlights the threat posed by the HIV/AIDS epidemic to global peace and security.
July 2000	UN Security Council adopts Resolution 1308 on the need to combat the spread of HIV/AIDS during peacekeeping operations.
July 2000	G8 Summit (Okinawa) commits to improving efforts to control HIV/AIDS and other infectious disease in selected countries.
April 2001	UN Secretary General Kofi Annan calls for establishment of a global fund on HIV/AIDS and health at the Organization for African Unity Summit (Abuja).
June 2001	UN Special Session on HIV/AIDS issues Declaration of Commitment on national strategies to address the spread of HIV/AIDS among uniformed personnel.
July 2001	G8 Summit (Genoa) confirms establishment of global fund with US$1 billion in contributions.
November 2001	G7 Health Ministers' Meeting agrees 'Ottawa Plan for improving health security' including the threat of bioterrorism.
March 2002 G7	Health Ministers' Meeting statement of agreed actions to improve the health security of its citizens.

---

industry, information industry and 'lifestyles' industry. Others have put forward proposals to create a system of global health cooperation (Sterky et al. 1996; Frenk and Sepulveda 1997; Raymond 1997; Institute of Medicine 1997).

Equally important has been an awareness of the issues that significantly challenge traditional approaches to health policy and development focused on the role of the state. While globalization had been extensively studied and debated since the 1970s in a number of fields, it was not until the mid 1990s that the subject began to be concertedly explored by scholars, policy makers and practitioners in the health field. Globalization has rapidly come to be recognized as one of the defining features of health policy in the early twenty-first century, led by such issues as emerging and re-emerging infectious diseases (ERIDs), environmental change, epidemiological and demographic trends, and technological developments. As a result, many voices have been united in their call for a global approach to health. What this means precisely, and what actions are needed in response, remains unclear.

The conceptual framework of this book seeks to take the above, sometimes divergent, voices beyond rhetorical or token mentions of global health. It is a framework that has been developed through wide-ranging reviews of the available empirical evidence on globalization and health, alongside ongoing discussions with health practitioners, policy makers and scholars. As defined above, globalization is a set of processes that are changing the nature of human interaction by intensifying those interactions across certain boundaries that have hitherto separated individuals and population groups from each other. These three types of boundary (spatial, temporal and cognitive) have become increasingly eroded and redefined, resulting in new forms of social organization and interaction across them.

Taking each of these in turn, and expanding upon them in subsequent chapters, the spatial dimension concerns changes to how we experience and perceive physical or territorially-based space. In broad terms, globalization is believed to be leading to a growing 'sense of the world as a single place' (Robertson 1992) due to increased travel, communication, trade and other shared experiences. This process of spatial globalization can be understood as occurring gradually over many centuries, from the migration of *Homo erectus* and *Homo sapiens* out of Africa, to the rise and fall of ancient civilizations, to the age of imperialism and the Industrial Revolution. Since the end of the Second World War, there has been an intensification and diversification of human contact across geographical space, enabled foremost by developments in mass transportation and communication technologies.

The resulting spatial changes have taken two forms. The first is a redefinition of existing territorially-based geographies, or the development of new forms of social geography. This is reflected in the continued political strength of nationalism in many parts of the world, with existing states fragmenting or combining into new states. The development of regionalism, through the European Union, North American Free Trade Agreement (NAFTA) and other regional initiatives, can be understood as a result of pressures to reorganize existing social and political space. Thus, there is evidence that globalization is reinforcing existing territorial boundaries, at the same time as creating new divisions within and across territorial spaces.

The second is what might be referred to as the 'death of distance' (Cairncross 1997) by which an increasing degree of social interaction is detached from territorial space. Scholte (2000: 46–7) writes that this 'deterritorialization' or growth of 'supraterritorial' relations between people is the defining feature of globalization, leading to 'far reaching change in the nature of social space'. Emails, conference calls, satellite television and virtual offices are all forms of social interaction that are independent of physical space. Similarly, global environmental change, foreign exchange trading and e-commerce operate without regard to territorial distance. Importantly, Scholte notes that this is a relative shift away from a world where social geography is entirely territorial, defined by sovereign states since the Treaties of Westphalia (1640), to one where nonterritorial geographies are emerging. Overall, the spatial dimension of globalization is creating diverse changes to the physical boundaries of human interaction. Geography continues to be a fundamental parameter for human societies, but there are unique and profound changes to how we perceive and experience physical space (Gottdiener 1994).

The temporal dimension of globalization concerns changes to the actual and perceived time in which human interaction takes place. Closely linked to the spatial dimension, reterritorialization or even deterritorialization of territorial geography is enabling the speeding up of many forms of human interaction. Such changes are perhaps most noticeable in communications. The invention and spread of telegraphy from the late 1830s across Europe, the US and Japan was central to burgeoning commercial and government activities, as well as the creation of a daily news service. The arrival of radio (known as wireless telegraphy) and telephony in the late nineteenth century brought new innovations that enabled communication across wider distances and larger numbers of people. The twentieth century brought the telex, satellite, facsimile, cellular or mobile telephone and, perhaps most significantly, the Internet, so that by the beginning of the twenty-first century much audio and visual communication has become virtually instantaneous across the globe. The application of these technologies, in turn, have transformed a wide range of human interactions – daily currency trading via worldwide computer systems totalled US$1.7 trillion daily in 1997, two-thirds of this trading for less than seven days (*The Economist* 1997). According to the so-called Moore's law, microchip density doubles every eighteen months, bringing greater memory capacity to computers. Gleick (1999:85) describes the change in communication speed in the following way:

> In a less connected time, any business deal based on an exchange of paperwork proceeded at a pace controlled by the mails – two, four, six, or more days between volleys. Then came universal overnight mail and its industrial-age children – in Federal Express jargon,

'expedited cargo', 'just-in-time delivery', 'high-speed premium transportation', and 'automating and streamlining the supply chain'. Federal Express sold its services for 'when it absolutely, positively has to be there overnight'. In the world before FedEx, when 'it' could not absolutely, positively be there overnight, it rarely had to. Now that it can, it must.

Although not quite as dramatic, developments in transportation technologies have accelerated social interaction in important ways. The building of the railways in the mid nineteenth century has given way to transoceanic steamships, automobiles, jet and supersonic aircraft and bullet trains. People move about the world in increased numbers, for greater distances and faster speeds. Almost anywhere on earth can now be reached within one day.

The cognitive dimension of globalization concerns changes to the creation and exchange of knowledge, ideas, norms, beliefs, values, cultural identities and other thought processes. How we think about ourselves and the world around us is being changed by globalization. The sources of these emerging thought processes are varied – the mass media, educational institutions, advertising agencies, think tanks, scientific bodies, consultancy firms, international organizations and 'spin doctors'. On the one hand, there is a greater sharing of thought processes across the world in the form of popular culture (such as Hollywood films, pop music, fashion), scientific research, and international norms and standards (for example human rights). On the other hand, there is strong resistance to the globalization of thought processes as expressed through anti-globalization protests against global corporations and resurgence of religious fundamentalism against 'western imperialism' (Beyer 1994).

As well as thought processes, globalization is having an impact on the process of knowledge creation. The universalization of the English language, spread of certain education theories and practices, funding patterns for research and development, and the adoption of intellectual property law internationally[6] raise implications for how and what knowledge is produced. While there is more intellectual activity than ever before,[7] there are concerns regarding its normative basis, ownership and commodification by certain vested interests, and appropriateness for the needs of local communities. In short, globalization is centrally about 'our mental frameworks – for example the way that we think about social institutions and forms of political authority in the brave new world of a globalising capitalism' (Gill 1997). Yet the apparent move towards a 'unified consciousness'[8] holds collective possibilities, as well as inherent contradictions.

Together, distinguishing among spatial, temporal and cognitive boundaries is a useful analytical framework for beginning to understand the diverse and complex changes that globalization may be bringing about. Using these three dimensions as a starting point, we can apply them to specific spheres of social interaction to identify the impacts of globalization. The spheres below are indicative, rather than comprehensive, and serve to separate out and organize seemingly disparate forces at play. The first is the economic sphere that can be described as concerning the production, distribution and consumption of wealth. The organizing principles for achieving this, in terms of inputs, modes of production and scale of operation are argued to be changing as a consequence of globalization. It is argued that we are moving towards a global economy by which there are larger economies of scale, greater exchange of goods, services and capital, and increased mobility of labour and other inputs. However this has been an uneven process, with some sectors (for example automobile, food) demonstrating strong globalizing features, with others less so.

Within the health literature, there has been a heavy focus on the economic sphere, notably the direct and indirect impacts of multilateral trade agreements (MTAs) on health. The conclusion of the Uruguay Round of the General Agreement of Tariffs and Trade (GATT)[9] in 1994, and the creation of the World Trade Organization (WTO) in 1995, led to concerns about inadequate protection of public health under specific MTA provisions notably the Agreement on Trade-Related Intellectual Property Rights (TRIPS) and the General Agreement on Trade in Services (GATS) (Navarro 1998; Zarilli and Kinnon 1998). Diseases transmittable by the trade of goods and services (that is foodborne diseases) have been given particular attention (Kaferstein et al. 1997). While some international agreements exist to deal with the health impacts of trade, such as the Agreement on the Application of Sanitary and Phytosanitary Measures and the *Codex Alimentarius*, the extent to which their stipulations have primacy over the rules of the WTO remains unclear (Fidler 1996). The 1997 ruling by the WTO on hormone-treated beef imported from the US into the European Union, in favour of American producers demonstrated that trade liberalization took precedence over public health protection where evidence of harmful health effects could not be readily proven. The ruling in favour of the Ethyl Corporation over the Canadian government, under the North American Free Trade Agreement (NAFTA), has added to these concerns. The more general effects of a globalizing economy, without sufficient protection of health and the environment, have attracted growing attention. Of particular concern is the lack of internationally agreed and enforced regulations on, *inter alia*, quality assurance, hygiene standards, labelling, marketing practices, the use of child labour, and the protection of occupational health and safety. Issues have also been raised by the so-called 'race to the bottom' in social welfare provision in those countries (often low-income countries) where governments compete for global trade and investment (Deacon et al. 1997).

The political sphere concerns the distribution and use of power. Because of globalizing forces, many writers argue that who holds power, the forms of power being wielded, and ways that power is being used are changing. This has led to discussion of the need for new forms of political representation such as global civil society and public–private partnerships, and emerging forms of authority towards global governance. In the health literature, less attention has been given to this sphere. A notable exception is Moran and Wood (1996) who describe four ways in which health policy is becoming more 'globalized': (a) changes to policy making whereby global networks among policy actors have developed, or global actors penetrate policy making in individual states; (b) implementation of health policy whereby health services or health care users migrate across national boundaries; (c) organization of production and supply of health products (such as equipment, drugs); and (d) the 'mindset' of national policy makers (for example health sector reform). This is a useful starting point for exploring globalization and health policy, but broader political issues beyond policy making warrant further consideration. This is discussed in greater detail in Chapter 6.

The sociocultural sphere concerns the collective activities, shared identities and traditions (such as values, beliefs, ideas), and support structures of societies. Perhaps the greatest impact of globalization on this sphere comes from the global reach of the mass media that, it is argued, is changing underlying cultural foundations. Some believe that globalization is contributing to new social identities across hitherto separated communities through, for instance, marketing and advertising, the Internet, and the popular television and film industry (Jameson and Miyoshi 1998). Despite a rich body of work on the globalization of the cultural sphere, the implications for health are yet to be fully adequately recognized. In 'AIDS as a Globalizing Panic', O'Neill (1990) considers HIV/AIDS as 'one of a number of panics of a political, economic, financial and "natural" sort to which the global order responds with varying strategies of crusade, sentimentality or force'. Such 'globalizing panics … rely heavily upon the media and television, newspapers, magazines, films and documentaries to specularize the incorporation of all societies into a single global system designed to overcome all internal division'. Altman (1996) examines the 'paradox of the apparent globalization of postmodern gay identities' or 'internationalization of a certain form of social and cultural identity' as a result of forces of global change which has led to homosexuality being increasingly interrogated. More broadly, Kalekin-Fishman (1996) explores the meaning and significance of ethical choices in health amid globalization, defined as a 'social process in which the constraints of geography on social and cultural arrangements recede and in which people become increasingly aware that they are receding'. Bettcher and Yach (1998) point to the need for a globalization of ethics given that many public health challenges transcend national boundaries.

The technological sphere can be broadly defined as the application of knowledge and skills for industry, commerce, the arts and science. Globalization is shaping what technologies are developed, as well as their use and dissemination through, for example, foreign trade and investment, research and development (R&D), education, and development assistance. On the one hand, globalization can be described as driven by technologies that enable processes of global change to occur. Transportation and communication technologies come readily to mind, but technologies influencing such diverse realms as food production and consumption, energy supplies and health care are also relevant. On the other hand, globalization is itself driving the development of particular technologies, access to them, and the ways in which they are used.

The environmental sphere concerns the natural and social surroundings within which people live and interact. Global change, both natural and anthropogenic, has attracted substantial attention and, indeed, environmental scientists and activists have led others in their appreciation of the interrelated nature of the emerging globalized world. It is perhaps most evident in the environmental sphere that what happens in one part of the world can have direct and indirect consequences for other parts of the world. In relation to health, the globalization of particular economic activities (such as unsustainable use of natural resources, toxic waste dumping), lifestyles (consumerism) and social structures (for example urbanization) has contributed to widespread environmental degradation both locally and globally. The anticipated impacts on health have generated a growing body of work. Gaining momentum after the UN Conference on Environment and Development in 1989, at which WHO was given responsibility for following up the health-related goals of Agenda 21, research has been initiated on the links between global environmental change and human health. The health implications of global climate change have received particular attention (McMichael and Haines 1997; Haines and McMichael 1997), including the anticipated epidemiological impacts on diseases such as malaria, cholera, schistosomiasis, yellow fever and Lyme borreliosis (Wilson et al. 1994; Murray and Lopez 1996; de Cock et al. 1995; Barthold 1996; Colwell 1996; Patz et al. 1996; Wise 1997). The problem of harmful transborder externalities created by industrial hazards and dumping of toxic waste is also being documented (Castleman and Navarro 1987; Castleman 1995).

1.4 Purpose and structure of the book

The purpose of this book is to provide an introduction to the emerging subject of global health. This volume is structured around the conceptual framework presented in Section 1.3 for understanding the links between globalization and health. Acknowledging the varying, and to a large extent, contested nature, of globalization, the conceptual framework offered here aims to help make heuristic sense of these links, but by no means is it a definitive one. There are more theoretically sophisticated frameworks available that delve more deeply into, for example, causal relationships between globalization and social change (Held et al. 1999; Scholte 2000). The framework of this book aspires only to be an analytically useful starting point to understand the shift from international to global health, the key issues raised by this shift, and how we should act to promote and protect the health of individuals and populations.

The book is organized along the three dimensions of globalization described above. Chapter 2 sets out the historical context of globalization and its impacts on health. This is followed by a discussion of each dimension of globalization in Chapters 3–5, illustrated with empirical examples of its implications for human health. Each chapter provides suggestions for further reading. The conclusions presented in Chapter 6 summarize key issues in global health to guide further research and policy action. Specific attention is given to how globalization is currently understood, what features are being given particular focus and, importantly, where there are gaps in present thinking and practice.

Table 1.1   The dimensions and spheres of global health

Dimensions/ Spheres	Spatial	Temporal	Cognitive
Economic	Transnational restructuring of production and exchange activities of health-related industries	Faster movement of infectious agents through intensified trade in plants and animals More rapid movement of new health interventions from laboratory to market	Proliferation of neoliberal-based health policies worldwide as part of health sector reform Global assertion of intellectual property rights over native plants, genomic codes, drugs
Political	Transnational mobilization of civil society groups concerned with health	Rapid response campaigning for health-related causes	Spread of support for concept of health as a human right
Sociocultural	New forms of identity emerging around shared health needs	Spread of fast-paced lifestyles and related physical and mental health conditions	Influence of global mass media on healthy lifestyles
Technological	Creation of new types of space through information and communication technologies	Ability to undertake disease surveillance and monitoring at a faster pace	Use of the Internet by governments, WHO, consultancy firms, research institutions, advertising companies to disseminate health-related information
Environmental	Spillover of environmental impacts (e.g. health effects of Chernobyl accident)	Accelerated depletion of natural resources Faster movement of genetic material worldwide	Spread of concept of sustainability to inform health policy

Source: Based on K. Lee (2000), 'Globalisation and health policy: A conceptual framework and research and policy agenda' in A. Bambas, H. Drayton eds, *Health and Human Development in the New Global Economy* (Washington DC: Pan American Health Organization): 15–41.

The book is intended to be accessible for those readers interested in either health or globalization. The latter, notably within the field of politics and international relations, shows a continued and surprising neglect of health issues among its voluminous works. Yet it is argued here that health issues offer examples to inform, illustrate and test ideas, concepts and theories that have been at the heart of scholarly and practical debates on globalization. The 'value-added' in this book is the insights that it provides from the health field, both conceptually and empirically, to understanding globalization. This book argues that the protection and promotion of human health must be an integral part of a form of globalization that is sustainable, equitable and socially just.

The second audience is students, scholars and practitioners in the health field. This book aims to draw insights from other fields grappling with the challenges of global change, in order to illuminate the challenges posed for human health. For example, cultural studies can offer insights into global trends in health sector reform and so-called lifestyle diseases. Political studies can provide ideas for the strengthening of global health governance. Economic analysis can shed light on trends in the structure of health-related industries and health care systems. Environmental studies can be drawn on to understand changes in the social and natural environments as broad determinants of health. And studies of technology can be used to understand the potential uses of information and communication systems for health promotion. At the same time, the book seeks to go beyond applying the insights of other fields for understanding global health issues. By drawing on other disciplines outside of the health field, theoretical and conceptual thinking could be brought to bear to understand and illuminate health issues and inform policy responses. Given these two rather different audiences that seldom come together in a concerted way, this book attempts to bridge this analytical and practical gap.

In seeking to reach both audiences, the book relies strongly on diverse and numerous examples. If it were presented in a restaurant, it would be a platter of starters that, while not perhaps filling in itself, provides a sufficient range of choice to stimulate one's appetite for further research and policy debate. Thus, the breadth of the book is admittedly wide-ranging, with less attention to in-depth analysis of the specific topic areas raised. While a necessary feature of such an introductory book, it also serves to demonstrate the fundamental ways that human health and globalization are intertwined.

2
Globalization and Health: A Historical Perspective

We are transient participants in this great, unfinished adventure.
A. J. McMichael, *Human Frontiers, Environments and Disease* (2001: 8)

2.1 Introduction

The historical timescale of when globalization began (and potentially ends), the pace at which it has evolved and spread, and the balance between forces of continuity and change, are among its most contested features. Undoubtedly, dating globalization is largely dependent on one's definition of the process. Scholte (1998: 17–18), for example, writes that globalization is 'a relatively recent event in world history', one that 'did not figure continually, comprehensively, intensely, and with rapidly increasing frequency in the lives of a large proportion of humanity until around the 1960s'. In contrast, Robertson (1992) dates globalization from the beginning of the fifteenth century from which it emerges in five distinct phases. Giddens (1990: 64) similarly describes the globalizing of modernity as a process of 'intensification of worldwide social relations which link distant localities in such a way that local happenings are shaped by events occurring many miles away and vice versa'. These processes are occurring over many centuries, embracing the establishment of the states system, rise of industrialism, and worldwide spread of capitalism. Still others take an even longer historical perspective, locating globalization with the migration of the *Homo* genus out of Africa some 1.6 million years ago.

The merit in these varying historical timescales depends on the aspect of globalization we are concerned with. If it is a complete history of human health, a return to the origins of the *Homo* genus over a period of one to two million years allows us to link patterns of health and disease with the evolutionary roots of human physical, behavioural and social adaptation. On the history of the modern world as constructed today, we might look back through several thousand years or so to the beginning of recorded history to help us understand how the health of populations has been intimately shaped by the formation of the states system, mercantilism and market capitalism. Finally, in order to appreciate the distinct challenges that the recent intensification of globalization holds for health, a historical perspective from the end of the Second World War is perhaps most appropriate.

The framework used in this chapter, and the book as a whole, is adapted from Held et al. (1999), a framework that fits well with the history of human health and disease. They describe forms of globalization in terms of four historical periods: pre-modern (before 1500), early modern (1500–1850), modern (1850–1945) and contemporary (from 1945 onwards). Each period is defined by 'spatio-temporal and organizational attributes of global interconnectedness' that characterize the distinct and changing nature of globalization over time. These attributes are extensity of global networks, intensity of global interconnectedness, velocity of global flows, and impact propensity of global interconnectedness (Table 2.1).

Using this framework, the aim of this chapter is to condense the rich tapestry of human history into sufficiently broad themes to illuminate how globalization, as it proceeds over many centuries, has impacted upon health. The first three periods are explored in this chapter in terms of the spatial, temporal and cognitive dimensions of globalization, drawing illustratively rather than comprehensively, on key historical events. The fourth period (from 1945 onwards) of contemporary globalization will be the subject of the other chapters of this book. In undertaking such an analysis, a broad range of sources are drawn upon to piece together what is admittedly a complex and, in many cases, fiercely disputed picture of the evolution of human societies. There are a substantial number of well-established works on the history of human health, but even these are limited by shortfalls in the quantity and quality of relevant data. The paucity of official records (for example for births, deaths, cause of death) before the nineteenth century in most countries, varying nomenclature, and subjective nature of accounts of medical conditions all pose challenges for scholars of medical history. Nonetheless, new scientific methods of research are continually being developed (such as DNA sequencing analysis, computer modelling, carbon dating) that will undoubtedly add to and

Table 2.1   Historical development of globalization

Period	Characteristics
Pre-modern (1000–1500)	• Spread of *Homo sapiens* to all major land areas except Antarctica • Shift from hunter-gatherer to agriculture-based communities • Ancient civilizations (e.g. China, Islam, Aztec) as separate and autonomous with limited trade and cultural flows between them • Fragmented political associations and overlapping authority structures in medieval Europe • Interregional globalization within Eurasia and the Americas • Political and military empires • Movements of peoples into uncultivated areas
Early modern (1500–1850)	• Initial European imperial expansionism into the Americas and Oceania during Age of Exploration/Discovery • Movement of Africans via the slave trade to the New World • Spread of world religions especially Christianity and Judaism • Formal creation of international society of states (Treaties of Westphalia, 1648) • Beginnings of diplomacy and regularization of interstate networks
Modern (1850–1945)	• Consolidation of international society of states and liberal democracies in Europe and United States • Spread of nationalism • Beginnings of global networks and cultural flows dominated by European powers • Creation of many new international organizations to provide stability and facilitate expansion of industrial capitalism • Rapid developments in transportation and communication technologies
Contemporary (1945–present)	• Worldwide states system overlaid by regional and global forms of regulation and governance • Decolonization of colonial territories • Global reach of transport and communication technologies • Degradation of natural environment • Growing transnational hierarchies of power and wealth • Emerging forms of global governance in the form of new transnational and nonterritorial forms of political agency and organization

Source: Adapted from D. Held, A. McGrew, D. Goldblatt and J. Perraton (1999), *Global Transformations, Politics, Economics and Culture* (Stanford: Stanford University Press).

revise our present knowledge, as well as open the door to alternative understandings.

Despite these imperfections, it is clear that health cannot be understood in isolation from wider historical forces at play including processes of globalization. Katz writes that 'an epidemic is as much the product of the sociological, geographical, and political factors of its time as is any other historical event' (Katz 1974: 422). More broadly speaking, McMichael (2001:2) writes that 'a population's profile of health and disease is essentially an expression of its social and physical environments'. The relationship between globalization and health is thus an intimate one. Globalization, in all its historical forms, is a core factor in the ups and downs of human health over time. In turn, the history of the human species is as much a story about the 'health' as the 'wealth' of nations. There is sheer drama to this story, a story that continues to unfold to the present day.

2.2 The evolution of human societies, health and disease before 1500

There is a well recognized and studied association between historical patterns of movement and settlement of peoples, their lifestyles, cultural practices, food sources, and corresponding patterns of health and disease. How human societies have evolved, from the earliest migrations by the *Homo* genus, continues to be a subject of ongoing scientific debate (Shreeve 1995). Developments in genome research since the late twentieth century have opened up the historical study of human populations through new knowledge and lines of enquiry. Current thinking holds that the *Homo* lineage originates in Africa, migrating beyond the continent to reach Dmanisi, Georgia, 1.7 million years ago and possibly Java, Indonesia even earlier. These earliest migrations (for example, of *Homo erectus, Homo habilis*) marked the starting point of a gradual process over many generations as hominids sought out food and other resources. The eventual spread of *Homo sapiens* to other continents occurred as part of this process, with concurrent waves of human migration out of Africa into the Middle East, Asia, Europe and beyond.

According to the 'Eve' hypothesis, our direct ancestors *Homo sapiens sapiens* evolved some 200,000 years ago in Africa, and began to migrate some 50,000 and 100,000 years ago from the continent. With superior intellectual capabilities, *Homo sapiens sapiens* gradually pushed out other hominid species, such as *Homo sapiens neanderthalensis,* to dominate Africa, Europe and Asia, as well as Australia, remote Pacific Islands and the Americas (Cann 2001). By between 10,000 and 4000 BC, modern humans were globally dispersed, occupying all the major land masses except Antarctica (Walker and Shipman 1996). Each biological evolution and social adaptation, beginning with the transition from living in trees to open grasslands, brought alterations to patterns of health and disease. Encounters with certain flora and fauna brought humans into contact with particular disease vectors and microbes. Changing sources and quantities of food led to certain nutritional benefits, as well as diet-related conditions (such as foodborne diseases, vitamin deficiencies). Conditions of habitation, such as density of living quarters and access to clean water and sanitation, affected proneness to infectious agents. And certain social behaviours either benefited (for example cooperative hunting) or harmed (for example, female infanticide) population health. The link between human migration and malaria is described in Box 2.1.

Cohen (1989: 17) notes two broad trends in the archaeological record of human societies – the gradual increase in overall size and density of human population, and the progressive displacement of smaller communities and political units by larger ones. Early prehistory 'band societies' of 30–50 individuals were hunter-gatherer societies exploiting wild sources of food within a given territory. Indeed, the hunting prowess of these societies led to local extinction of large-bodied game animals which, in turn, drove humans to migrate further afield in search of new prey. The health status of these paleolithic hunter-gatherers was, on the whole, relatively good despite comparatively short lifespans. Also, as populations moved into more temperate climates, disease organisms that thrive in tropical zones became less important. The diseases afflicting these relatively small and mobile societies became either parasitic organisms, caused by bodily contact, plants and other animals for their continuity (for example rabies, toxoplasmosis, haemorrhagic fevers, anthrax), or slow-acting and chronic diseases such as yaws and herpes (McNeill 1976: 32–3).

Eventually, the widespread depletion of big game forced further adaptations in early human societies in the search for new food sources, the most significant being the domestication of plants and animals. Such was the success of food production that it opened the way for substantial and rapid increases in population, resulting in population densities ten to twenty times greater than in hunting societies only a few hundred years before (McNeill 1976: 43). The collective living of hundreds, as opposed to tens, of individuals and their close

Box 2.1   A brief history of malaria and the evolution of human societies

The historical distribution of malaria is an interesting example of the close link between changing social and natural environments, and patterns of disease. As McMichael (2001: 78–85) describes, the evolutionary origins of malaria take us back 50 million years when the single-celled protozoan organism *Plasmodium falciparum* first infected our ancestral primate species. The *Plasmodium* genus infected reptiles and birds during the Mesozoic period, and began to infect mammals once dinosaurs became extinct. By the early Tertian period, malaria parasites began to infect primates. The complex life cycle of the parasite that has evolved has created a triangular relationship of plasmodia, mosquito and human. Today, four species of plasmodium infect humans, three from simian origins (*vivax, malariae* and *ovale*) and the other from birds (*falciparum*).

Malaria spread to other parts of the world, and evolved further, with the migration of the *Homo* genus, plasmodium and anopheline mosquitoes out of Africa. This was limited somewhat by the plasmodium's need for temperatures between 20–24 degrees centigrade depending on the particular species. As world and regional temperatures waxed and waned with periods of glaciation, affecting the creation of suitable habitats, so too did the distribution of malaria. The current Holocene interglacial from around 10,000 years ago allowed various malaria parasites to spread further north. These changes to the natural environment (temperature, precipitation and vegetation) were accompanied by human-induced changes through forest clearing, farming practices and building of irrigation systems during the Neolithic period around 4000 years ago (de Zulueta 1994: 8). Falciparum malaria thus became established in African populations, but remained a rare infection in Greece during the fifth century BC. The refractoriness of tropical strains of *P. falciparum* to infect European vectors also acted as a barrier for many centuries. However, *P. vivax* spread northwards during the ensuing five centuries, from the shores of the Mediterranean into most parts of Asia. Increased migration and trade in the Mediterranean region and adjacent lands during Hellenistic and early Roman times then spread the parasite to southern Europe. Malaria was not a serious problem during the height of the Roman Empire until two new mosquito vectors (from North Africa and South Asia) became established in the Mediterranean region (McMichael 2001: 80–1). The subsequent spread of the disease to other parts of Europe, including the British Isles, Sweden and Russia, occurred during the decline of the Roman Empire. Further deforestation for agriculture added to the establishment of favourable habits for breeding mosquitoes (de Zulueta 1987:203).

A similar story can be found in Asia where the drop in temperatures during the last glaciation was less marked, offering an opportunity for the disease to spread to northern latitudes faster in that region. The Indus civilization suffered terribly from malaria, quite likely as a result of the depletion of riverine forests for baking mud bricks. This environmental change, in turn, may have affected the behaviour of the *Anopheles stephenisi*, which became the most effective vector in urban conditions, contributing to the

---

Box 2.1   continued

end of the civilization in the middle of the second millennium BC. Malaria spread by ships from the Indian subcontinent to ancient Mesopotamia (modern-day Iraq) where the local mosquito *A. pulcherrimus* was a poor vector for the parasite. It was not until the spread of *A. stephenisi* to the region that malaria increased, a mosquito that remains the most important vector in Iraq today (de Zulueta 1994: 10).

The history of malaria for the next centuries is less well known although it is clear that the disease continued to be spread through human activity. Based on molecular genetic studies, and the fact that it would have been difficult for the parasite to reach the Americas in prehistoric times, particularly during the last glaciation (de Zulueta 1987: 196), it is widely agreed that malaria is an Old World disease. There is strong evidence that *P. vivax* was introduced into Latin America in the early sixteenth century, benefiting from the widespread anopheline mosquito in the region. *P. falciparum* was then spread from West Africa to the Americas via the slave trade. Australia remained free of malaria until 1849 when European settlers introduced it. During the early twentieth century, the replacement of vast tracts of jungle by rubber plantations to support the burgeoning rubber trade led to a major increase in malaria transmission via *A. maculatus* mosquito. At the same time, the first noticeable decline of malaria occurred in Europe during the nineteenth century as a result of new agricultural practices and social conditions. Overall, the history of malaria is intimately connected to human history. As de Zulueta (1987: 203) writes, 'Man, more than Mother Earth, was the one to change the distribution of malaria, from the dawn of civilization until the present time'.

---

contact in one location brought profound changes to their health status. Initially, they were more vulnerable to local parasites. Permanent dwellings attract vermin – rodents, insects – and the diseases carried by these vectors. A wide variety of intestinal parasites such as worms could now also move from host to host via faecal matter or contaminated water supplies. With the development of animal husbandry, diseases arising from the closer vicinity of animals (zoonosis) added to the ailments of early societies.

Nonetheless, the continued rapid growth of human populations during this early period suggests that diseases did not take a heavy toll until communities reached the size that allows epidemic diseases to develop and spread. For example, it is estimated that a population of 200,000 people is needed to sustain a measles outbreak. The capacity to sustain larger communities was predicated on the community's capacity to provide adequate food, water, sanitation and housing. The development of irrigation systems to further increase food supplies, for example, correspondingly created favourable breeding and living conditions for vectors of certain diseases in tropical climates such as schistosomiasis (snail) and malaria (mosquito). In short, continued alterations to the natural environment, coupled with increasingly dense populations, brought changes to patterns of health and disease.

Eventually, as societies grew larger still to form towns and cities, migration and trade among different communities steadily developed. With increased population mobility came the exchange of health-influencing factors such as infectious agents, food sources and cultural practices. McNeill (1976) writes that the historical patterns of bodily contact and human disease are joined by three major events: (a) the linking of China, India and the Mediterranean by land and sea early in the Christian era; (b) the spread of the Mongol empire during the thirteenth century; and (c) the beginning of European exploration from the fifteenth century. Perhaps the most significant examples were the plague (bubonic and pneumonic) epidemics that visited Asia and Europe periodically, killing up to half of the affected population in some places. Indeed, plague is often cited as an early example of the increasingly globalized nature of health whereby the health status on one continent is substantially affected by events on another continent (Box 2.2).

While the bacterial infection that causes plague was little understood in the fourteenth century, what was soon realized was the close link between the disease and trade with Asia. It was the epidemic of the 1370s that led to the development of the first system of maritime quarantine aimed at preventing the importation of the disease. Other European countries followed suit. For overland travellers, a type of health passport was created that would certify their plague-free status. The need to administer these measures required an efficient bureaucracy and boards of health were formed across many countries. Indeed, as Carmichael (1997:63) writes, plague was 'an undeniable stimulus to the growth of the modern bureaucratic state'. The last great epidemic occurred in Marseilles, France, in 1722 (resulting in over 50,000 deaths) which led to redoubled efforts to strengthen quarantine measures. This included the establishment of a 1500-mile *cordon sanitaire* from the Balkans to north of the Danube. Measures were taken to restrict the cloth trade with the Middle East, given suspicions that the disease was somehow transmitted through it. The line of guard houses administering the quarantine, however, did little to stop the spread of plague, instead redirecting trade and eventually the disease itself to central Russia during 1770–71. As discussed in Chapter 6, these efforts

---

Box 2.2   The intercontinental migration of plague

Plague is caused by a bacterial infection of fleas, *Yersinia pestis*, which was carried by rodents from the central Asian plains across Asia and Europe between the fourteenth and eighteenth centuries. It is believed that the plague bacillus was brought to Italy in 1348 from Asia by ship, either by arriving merchants or returning crusaders. The local brown rat, *Rattus rattus*, soon became infected with the bacillus that, in turn, passed the disease onto human populations living in the densely populated cities and towns of the Middle Ages. Patterns of disease also suggest that *Y. pestis* became endemic among local rodent colonies until the seventeenth century. When winters arrived, and the rat population began to wane due to their own high levels of mortality, the main mode of transmission changed from bacillus–rats–human (vector-borne) to human–human (airborne). This change from bubonic to pneumonic plague had devastating consequences over the next several years, as the plague returned at least four times to most Mediterranean cities. From Europe and Asia, plague then spread to the New World from the late fifteenth century via explorers, traders and migrants. At the turn of the twentieth century, the disease reached California by ship, causing an epidemic infection in San Francisco. It then spread to wildlife where it established a reservoir and continues to this day to cause occasional outbreaks upon contact between the flea-carrying hosts, such as squirrels, and human populations. There remains speculation as to why plague disappeared from Europe, the only continent today that has no naturally occurring *Y. pestis* in rodents. The effectiveness of maritime quarantine may have limited the number of infected rats and fleas reaching western Europe. Alternatively, the development of global oceanic trade may have opened up alternative trade routes to Asia. Others suggest that regional climate changes, resulting in cooler temperatures, have led to changes in the occurrence of rodent populations.

Source: Ziegler P. (1969), *The Black Death* (London: Collins).

---

at exclusion simply served to drive the disease elsewhere, an important lesson when diseases become even more globalized by the twentieth century.

Population mobility is not the only factor that has influenced the spread of pathogens across territorial distances. Migratory birds are the natural hosts of many arboviruses. The vectors of such diseases are ticks and mites that infest nests and infect chicks. The arthropods themselves or the virus is transported via migrating birds travelling between breeding and feeding grounds. There are many known examples of risks to human health arising from bird migration. It is believed, for example, that viruses transported by migratory birds to and from the Arctic region posed a major health hazard for humans migrating from Asia to the Americas, as well as possibly causing the extinction of some native animal species. Long-distance dispersal of the *Ixodes dammini* tick by migratory birds off the New England coast (Smith et al. 1996), and *Ixodes persulcatus* tick in Japan (Miyamoto et al. 1997; Ishiguro et al. 2000) is thought to be responsible for the movement of Lyme disease from endemic to non-endemic areas. A recent example is West Nile virus, a disease first recorded in the New World in 1999 where the outbreak led to 62 cases and seven deaths in New York. Ornithophilic mosquitoes are the primary vectors of the virus in the Old World, and migrant birds are believed to be the main introductory or amplifying host. As such, there is the potential for outbreaks throughout the western hemisphere (Rappole et al. 2000) originating from such far-flung locations as Madagascar. Similar studies on Sinbis (SIN) virus in Australia (Sammels et al. 1999), flaviviruses in Europe (Draganescu et al. 1975), and water birds in the distribution and circulation of influenza viruses suggests a highly complex relationship between human disease and the natural environment. As we shall see in Chapter 3, the extent to which human activity has impacted on the environment is an important factor in the spread of certain diseases.

The beginnings of spatial and temporal changes to patterns of health and disease, as described above, were accompanied by changes in thinking about health. The common perception of the causes of disease in many societies centred on divine forces that dole out rewards or punishments according to some moral framework. For example, during the plague epidemics of the 1340s and 1350s, the disease was seen among Europeans as a sign of God's displeasure with sinful humanity, and hence the need for order and redemption (Carmichael 1997:60). In Asia and Europe, what scientific explanations there were focused on astrological origins of disease, the disjunction of the planets and other heavenly spheres, or imbalances in the composition of matter or energies within the human body.

While this glance at the pre-modern period of globalization is unavoidably cursory, we can see that important foundations were laid for the changes brought by ensuing periods. The history of human health and disease is clearly a global story with origins in Africa following the migration of the *Homo* genus, then embracing increasingly larger parts of the world in a complex but interrelated evolutionary story. The health challenges encountered by the human species, as it struggled to survive and thrive, came from both natural (for instance glaciation) and human-induced (such as agricultural practices) changes to the environment. With evolutionary success, and the emergence of larger communities, so-called 'crowd diseases' played an especially important role in limiting the size of communities until the nineteenth century. Indeed, human population size remained relatively small until quite recently because of repeated extinctions and founder events (Cann 2001:1747). The precise details of this period of prehistory and early history continue to be revealed through new paleoanthropological discoveries. What is clear is that, with the arrival of Europeans in the Americas, life and death would never be the same.

2.3 The global health impact of European exploration from 1492

> *For the natives, they are neere all dead of small Poxe, so as the Lord hathe cleared our title to what we possess.*
>
> John Winthrop, first governor of Massachusetts Bay Colony, 1634
> (as quoted in Crosby 1986: 208)

> *The colony of a civilized nation which takes possession, either of waste country, or of one so thinly inhabited, that the natives easily give place to the new settlers, advances more rapidly to wealth and greatness than any other human society.*
>
> Adam Smith, *An Inquiry into the Nature and Causes of the Wealth of Nations* (1776)

There remains much in dispute about the migration of the human species to the Americas. In broad terms, the Americas were inhabited by humans at least 20,000, and possibly up to 50,000 years ago, crossing from Siberia to Alaska before migrating east and southwards. Within a few thousand years, humans had spread throughout North and South America. Much later, about 10,000 years ago, the Inuit people arrived in northern North America. Even later, about 4000–5000 years ago, a further wave of immigrants brought tribes to the Pacific northwest (the Haida, the Athapaskan) and southwest US (Navajo). The question of whether there was human contact between the peoples of the Americas and other continents before 1492 remains a subject of intense study. The populations of the Americas remained relatively isolated with the possible exception of current-swept arrivals from Kyushu, Japan to Ecuador over 5000 years ago, bringing with them pottery and, more contentiously, hookworm (Desowitz 1997). Nonetheless, pre-Columbian contact was a rarity. Furthermore, uniquely American species of flora and fauna, along with microbes and parasites, evolved during this period.

From the late fifteenth century, European (notably Spanish, Portuguese, British and French) explorers began a process, leading up to the present-day, of bringing together parts of the world hitherto largely separate – what many writers see as the historical roots of present-day globalization. This contact between the so-called 'Old' and 'New' worlds is admittedly a Eurocentric perspective. Many exchanges among non-European peoples preceded this period. The Chinese explorer Cheng Huo preceded European exploration by a century but these forays were discontinued by the Chinese emperor as undesirable (Benyon and Dunkerley, 2000: 7). More generally, as described above, human migration across continents has been a continual process, with concurrent waves of migrants moving about the globe. While not denying the importance of these earlier exchanges, from a human health perspective, Columbus's arrival in the Americas marks an important turning point in two ways.

First, globalization as presently manifest is a world order dominated by western societies. This book seeks to trace back the trajectory of the current and particular forms of globalization we have today, warts and all, to understand its health impacts. Second, scholars of the history of health and disease often return to 1492 as a defining event. Until the late fifteenth century, as Hays (1998) writes, 'Humans on different continents, and their accompanying parasites, had a period of separate evolution.' Similarly, Grmek's (1969 as cited in Berlinguer 1992) concept of 'pathocenosis' is useful here to describe the whole complex of pathological conditions that exist in a given population in a specific period. In the Old World, Europe and Asia experienced a continuous exchange of disease, with an integration of viral reservoirs between 500 BC and AD 1200. A completely different pathocenosis evolved in the Americas because of the limited movement of people to and from those continents (McNeill 1976).

This isolation ended with the Age of Discovery that brought an unprecedented 'movement of a wide assortment of animals, insects, and parasitic microorganisms' across continents. The health impact was a consequence of exchanges of food sources, cultural and social practices and, most immediately and dramatically, pathogens. The latter derived from the fact that populations in the Americas were hitherto unexposed to diseases that had taken their toll on other continents over many thousands of years. Biologically isolated from the Old World, Native Americans were highly vulnerable to diseases such as amoebic dysentery, chickenpox, diphtheria, German measles (rubella), influenza, measles, mumps, scarlet fever, smallpox, trachoma, typhoid fever, whooping cough and plague, all thought to have been transported by Europeans to the New World. The results were 'virgin soil epidemics' of very high morbidity and mortality, especially among the young adult population (Crosby 1972; McNeill 1976).

The actual size of the pre-Columbian American population remains contested, given poor written records, limited archaeological data, and the use of different methods of population projection. Estimates for North America range from two to 18 million (Dobyns 1966), and for the entire hemisphere from ten to 90–112 million. In general, it is agreed that the American population in the fifteenth century was similar to that of Europe, numbering between 50 and 100 million people (Hays 1998:72; Ellwood 2001). However, while Europe experienced rapid population growth during the sixteenth century, the Americas experienced a sudden decline of 50–90 per cent. McNeill (1976: 215) cites the change in population size between pre- and post-Columbian periods as between 20:1 and 25:1. Berlinguer (1992: 1408) describes this as 'the greatest demographic tragedy in history'.

While the exact causes of the decline in population remain disputed, it is acknowledged that infectious diseases introduced by Europeans played a key role. In some cases, diseases preceded the arrival of European settlers by decades or even tens of decades, spread inland along trade routes by native populations to devastate local communities. A notable example is the Inca which numbered around 14 million in the early sixteenth century. Smallpox arrived in the late 1520s and, within a few years the population was reduced by 30–50 per cent. Other epidemics followed including measles (1531), plague or typhus (1546–8), measles again (1556–8), and then smallpox, measles and typhus all at once (1585–91). Thus, when the Spanish explorer Francisco Pizarro arrived in 1532, he found a decimated and demoralized people whom he was able to conquer with relative ease (Roberts 1989).

The flow of pathogens occurred in other directions as well. The search for the riches of the Orient continued to motivate European explorers. Captain Cook's travels to Australasia during the eighteenth century brought a similar devastation of local populations through disease. The First Fleet arrived in Australia in 1788, and one year later a smallpox epidemic was raging among the Aborigines, eventually killing as much as one-third of the population. The disease returned three further times during the nineteenth century (Crosby 1986: 206).

Interestingly, human diseases of Australasia and the Americas do not seem to have been exported on a substantial level to the rest of the world. Perhaps the most notable, and still controversial, exception is syphilis. The complex bacteriology of the disease includes the fact that there are several species of bacterium *Treponema* that, in turn, are responsible for several distinct diseases including yaws, pinta and venereal syphilis (*Treponema pallidum*). The story of syphilis remains a highly contested but illuminating one for understanding the global migration of pathogens. There is much support for the Columbian theory of syphilis, namely that it was exported from the New World from 1492 to wreak devastation on Europe and Asia. Hays (1998) argues that no clinical descriptions of such a disease exists in European or Asian writing before the 1490s. Then, during the sixteenth century, writers in Spain, Germany, Italy, Egypt, Persia (Iran), India, China and Japan all describe a 'pox' that they had never seen before (Crosby 1972: 124). Furthermore, studies of skeletal remains by paleopathologists have not yielded syphilitic bone damage in the Old World (as found in pre-Columbian America). Clinical evidence, as well as the initial virulence of the epidemic, characteristic of a non-immune population, also supports the Columbian thesis.

Syphilis is thus thought to have first appeared in Europe in Italy in the mid 1490s in time to meet the invasions by the armies of Charles VIII of France during 1494–95. Soldiers were major conduits of disease, living in squalid conditions, highly mobile and usually ill-disciplined. As soldiers of fortune, recruited from many countries, they dispersed widely after conflicts to spread whatever infections they had acquired to other populations. Syphilis was reported throughout Europe, the Middle East and North Africa by 1499, and in China by 1509. The crew of Vasco da Gama are believed to have introduced the disease to India during their voyage of 1498. Although the disease spread without discrimination among social classes, afflicting some of the most prominent figures of the day such as Henry VIII, who is believed to have suffered from syphilis from 1509 to his death in 1547, and Ivan IV of Russia, similarly afflicted from 1533 to the end of his life in 1584, the disease carried much stigma. Terms to describe the disease – the French disease, Polish pox, Naples disease, German pox, ulcer of Canton – reflected this stigma but also its close association with foreigners. Again, this suggests the disease was newly imported.

Another important exchange that took place during this period, which had significant health impacts, was the trade in plants and animals. Before the sixteenth century, cultivated plants were generally restricted to the continents of their origin. Different patterns of agriculture emerged in the eastern and western hemispheres and, as such, almost entirely different groups of food plants were cultivated in pre-Columbian times. Given so few domesticated animals, Native Americans produced some of the most important food plants (including maize, beans, and potatoes).

In Europe, one of the major spurs behind Spanish and Portuguese explorers as they set sail in the late fifteenth century was the lucrative spice trade. As the Ottoman Turkish Empire controlled an increasing number of strategic trading routes to Asia, European countries sought alternative links to the spices of the 'Indies'. It was this search for the riches of the east that inadvertently brought Spanish ships to the Caribbean islands in the late 1490s, and which then accelerated the globalization of foodstuffs. Among the most important cultivated plants to be taken back to Europe, as well as to Africa and Asia, was maize. Easily cultivated in different climates, high-yielding, quick-growing and nutritional, maize was eagerly accepted by farmers. Indeed, such was the enthusiasm for this new food among many of the peoples of the Old World that pellagra, a disease resulting from deficiencies in vitamin C and nicotinic acid, began to appear. The disease was virtually unknown in the Americas because maize was balanced with other foods such as beans and vegetables (Tannahill 1973: 203–6). Other foodstuffs traded during the sixteenth century were much welcomed in Europe by a relatively ill-nourished populace and their arrival is believed to be critical to the further expansion of European populations from this period onwards. At the same time, the spread of food crops of American origin to Africa, notably maize and manioc, gradually improved diets on that continent and allowed an increase in population size (Table 2.2).

The decimation of Native American populations within a hundred years of Columbus's arrival, coupled with aspirations by Europeans to exploit the resources of the New World, soon meant a major labour shortage. With the unavailability of Native Americans to serve as labourers and servants (willing or otherwise), Europeans looked elsewhere to address this labour shortage. Morally, this was resolved by the Papal Bull of 1493 which drew a spiritual division between the European and non-European world, along with the souls of its peoples. Pope Alexander VI decreed West Africa to Portugal, and this opened the way for the largest transoceanic migration of any people up to that point in history – the transatlantic slave trade. According to analysis by Eltis et al. (1999), it is estimated that around 35,000 transatlantic slave

Table 2.2   Forms of human societies and patterns of health and disease

Type of Society	Features	Patterns of health and disease
Prehistory band society	Paleolithic period Nomadic Small size (30–50 individuals) Hunter-gatherers	1. Parasitic diseases not dependent on human host – rabies, tularemia, toxoplasmosis, haemorrhagic fevers, leptospirosis, brucellosis, anthrax, salmonellosis, gangrene, botulism, tetanus, trichinosis, tapeworms, staphylococcal infections, trypanosomiasis, tick-borne viral diseases 2. Chronic infections – Yaws, bacterial infections, herpes
Early human settlements (village)	Neolithic period Sedentary Agrarian Several hundred individuals Change natural environment Permanent dwellings Refuse and waste	1. Diseases from parasites in local soil and water – hookworm, schistosomiasis, malaria, onchocerciasis 2. Vector-borne diseases – yellow fever, dengue fever, encephalitis, bubonic plague, malaria 3. Airborne diseases – influenza 4. Fecal-oral infections – ascarid worms
Human settlements (towns and cities)	Several thousand individuals Intensified farming Specialization of skills and roles Increased trade and migration between societies Hierarchical social structure	1. Parasitic diseases transmitted from person to person 2. Fecal-oral diseases – worms, intestinal protozoa, bacteria, cholera, shigella 3. Vector-borne diseases 4. Airborne diseases – tuberculosis 5. Epidemic diseases (acute and short duration in human host) – bubonic plague, influenza, measles, mumps, rubella, smallpox, rhinovirusis, diphtheria, whooping cough, streptococcal bacteria

Source: Adapted from Cohen (1989), *Health and the Rise of Civilization* (New Haven: Yale University Press), chapter 4.

ship voyages were made between 1595–1866, bringing ten million arrivals to the Americas. Ninety per cent of the slaves were sent to the tropical regions of the Americas where they were used to mass produce export crops such as sugar, coffee, cotton, rice and tobacco (Crosby 1972: 213). The trade established a triangular relationship whereby European capital bought slaves in Africa, the slaves were shipped from Africa to the Americas, and the fruits of their labour were shipped back to Europe and beyond for consumption. It was a highly profitable arrangement for the slave traders and merchants classes.

Health is a key component of the story behind the slave trade, as well as the consequences of that trade for the world's populations. The slave trade introduced additional diseases to the Americas including malaria, yellow fever, filariasis, hookworm and schistosomiasis. Hence, the first epidemic of yellow fever in the New World is believed to have occurred in 1648 in the Yucatan and Cuba after *Aedes aegypti*, most probably carried in the water casks of ships from West Africa, became established in places with temperatures above 72°F (22°C). Once this species of mosquito found its niche in the local ecosystem, yellow fever reached epidemic proportions. While yellow fever, malaria and other African diseases affected Europeans and Native Americans alike, coming on the coat tails of European diseases, they exacted an especially heavy toll on the local populations (McNeill 1976: 213–15). Although African slaves enjoyed greater immunity from such diseases, making them even more desirable as workers, high mortality rates resulted from other causes. Under appalling conditions of transport from West Africa, many died prior to and during the long ocean voyage. Gastrointestinal disorders, ill treatment by slave owners and difficult working conditions took a further toll.

An important aspect of the globalization of health during this period was the beginnings of a global trade in addictive substances beginning with tobacco. Two species of tobacco plant, *Nicotiana rustica* and *Nicotiana tobacum*, were dispersed by Native Americans around 8000 years ago. Tobacco was introduced to Europeans in 1492, with Columbus writing in his diary that the local people carried 'a firebrand in the hand, and herbs to drink the smoke thereof, as they are accustomed'. The use of tobacco spread quickly among the Spanish settlers, and by 1571 the practice had spread to nearly all parts of Europe. A lucrative and substantial trade sprang up, with tobacco even becoming a means of currency in some parts of the colonies because of its coveted value. Imports of tobacco to England rose rapidly to become the leading item of commerce, from 60,000 pounds weight in 1622 to

20 million pounds annually by the end of the seventeenth century. Importantly, the production and trade of tobacco was enabled by, as well as supportive of, the colonization of the region, the flourishing slave trade and the emerging mercantile system. For example, because tobacco exhausted the soil of its nutrients after three years, new land continually needed to be cultivated. This drove Europeans to acquire more and more land from Native Americans, often under dubious terms.

The use of other addictive substances also has origins during this period. Crude opium, alone or dissolved in some liquid such as alcohol (laudanum), was brought to North America by European settlers and explorers. It is reported that Benjamin Franklin regularly took laudanum for pain relief late in his life, as did the poet Samuel Taylor Coleridge who had a lifelong addiction. Other drugs had been used for millennia in their natural form. Drugs such as cocaine and morphine, for example, were only available in coca leaves or poppy plants that were chewed, dissolved in alcoholic beverages or taken in a way that diluted the active ingredient (Musto 1991: 20). The beginnings of the trade in coffee and tea can also be included in this context, both luxury goods that were highly prized for their mild stimulant effect.

This period in the history of global health can be summarized as one of profound importance for the bringing together of diverse population groups, along with other forms of life, that were hitherto separate in evolutionary terms. From Columbus's arrival in 1492, the way was open for varied forms of human interaction that would influence patterns of health and disease in the Old and New Worlds. As McNeill (1976: 216) writes, 'in the first centuries after ships began to ply the oceans of the earth and united all the coastlines of the world into a single intercommunicating network, the process of homogenization of disease distribution involved expansion of some diseases onto new ground.' This set the foundations for the next phase of globalization as defined by the onset of the Industrial Revolution.

2.4   The global health dimensions of the Industrial Revolution (1750–1919)

If feces were fluorescent, the whole world would glow at night.

(Desowitz 1997:224)

The Industrial Revolution was a period of rapid progress, not only in the economic sphere, but across a wide range of human endeavour.

The social, cultural, political and technological changes brought about had profound impacts, initially in Europe but eventually worldwide. The great wealth generated by the Industrial Revolution led to steady improvements in quality of life for many through increased trade, employment opportunities and scientific advances. For millions of others, however, the decline of the agricultural sector, rapid urbanization, and shifting labour markets meant much upheaval. Throughout this period of globalization, the impacts on health were a central part of the story.

One defining feature of the Industrial Revolution was the demographic shifts in terms of the movement of people within and across countries. Populations expanded significantly during this period in many parts of the world, with particularly rapid growth in rural parts of Europe. Between 1750 and 1850 Europeans increased from 20 per cent to 23 per cent of the world's population. Importantly, this growth was accompanied by fundamental social change – what Doyal (1979: 49) describes as 'the beginnings of the transition from feudalism to capitalism [that] had savage effects on life (and death) in the countryside'. The development of so-called 'scientific agriculture' increased food yields through crop rotation, use of fertilizers and mechanization, but also dramatically reduced the demand for rural workers.

The result was large-scale migration to towns and cities during the eighteenth century and onwards, followed by migration abroad. Faced with low wages, high unemployment and widespread poverty, many set their sights on the New World. Thus began the largest transoceanic migration of people in history. European emigration to the Americas increased sharply during the nineteenth century. Between 1851 and 1960, 61 million Europeans migrated to other continents, 45 million by 1924 to the Americas. An additional factor was the potato famine of the mid 1840s. The potato was introduced into Ireland in the 1540s and subsequently became the staple (and often sole) food of much of the population. The potato blight (caused by egg-shaped disease spores) was spread from the northeast coast of North America in 1840 by ship to Europe in 1845. The disease resulted in famine throughout Europe, with particularly devastating impact on Ireland (Cohen 1996). The crisis led to mass emigration of the Irish to the growing industrial towns of England and the US, increasing from 60,000 before 1845 to 250,000 by 1851 (Tannahill 1973: 291). The arrival of the steamship and railroad further facilitated this mass migration of people between continents.

The health impacts of these major changes were also significant. One positive effect was the improved availability of a wider variety of foodstuffs through trade, at least to those who could afford to buy them. As plantations were established throughout the European colonial territories, products such as tea, coffee, wheat and sugar were shipped back to the Old World. Food preservation techniques also improved, expanding the range of products that could be traded long distances. The invention of canning around 1812 was a major advance, enabling foodstuffs to be safely preserved for long periods of time. By the 1860s bulk shipments of such canned goods as salmon became a lucrative business. In the 1830s the first ice-making machines were patented, eventually enabling fresh fruit and vegetables from around the world to be shipped. While the principles of sterilization had not yet been discovered, condensation of milk by adding sugar to inhibit bacterial growth was successful. The 1870s to 1890s saw the opening up of many colonized territories for mass meat production. In the US, the Great Plains were cleared of buffalo to accommodate large cattle ranches, a practice repeated in Australia, Canada and parts of South America. The scientific understanding of diet, notably the importance of vitamins, was also advanced during this period. Dutch investigation of beriberi[1] led to the scientific discovery of vitamins in the late 1880s, and marked the beginning of understanding diseases due to vitamin deficiencies. All of these developments led to fundamental changes in the diets of people worldwide through alterations in agricultural practices, continued migration of plants and animals (Table 2.3), and availability of foodstuffs.

While some health gains were achieved by improvements in diet, new risks emerged during the Industrial Revolution. Foremost was the threat from infectious disease, a disproportionate threat to disadvantaged individuals and population groups. In the rapidly growing towns and cities of Europe, the lack of accompanying infrastructure to provide clean water and sanitation, adequate housing and basic health care created ideal conditions for so-called 'crowd diseases' to occur and spread. The squalor of nineteenth-century urban life was worsened by the mass migration of people described above, from rural to urban areas, as well as from military conflict and migration abroad. Added to this were striking inequalities in socioeconomic status, the widespread use of child labour, and the lack of any formal system of social security.

It is unsurprising, therefore, that the history of the nineteenth century is one defined by vast inequalities and great epidemics. This is well illustrated by the history of cholera. For many centuries cholera was confined to the riverine areas of the Indian subcontinent. In the

Table 2.3   The geographical origins of selected cultivated food plants and animals

Americas	avocado, beans (butter, French, frijole, haricot, kidney, lima, navy, sieva, snap, string), Brazil nuts, cocoa, guava, maize, manioc (cassava), papaya, peanut, peppers (capsicum), pineapple, potato, pumpkin, squash, sweet potato, tapioca, tomato, turkeys, vanilla
	fowl
Europe	barley, cabbage, carrot, citrus fruits, garlic, honey, oats, onions, peach, plum, rye, sugar beet, turnip, wheat
	cattle, chickens, goats, honeybees, pigs, sheep
Africa	millet, sorghum
	guinea fowl
Asia	banana, cardamom, cinnamon, cloves, coconut, ginger, pepper, rice, saffron, sugar, tea
	pig (white), water buffalo

Sources: Compiled from R. Tannahill, *Food in History* (Harmondsworth: Penguin, 1973);
A. W. Crosby, *The Columbian Exchange, Biological and Cultural Consequences of 1492*
(Westport, Conn.: Greenwood Press, 1972), chapter 5; and A. W. Crosby, *Ecological
Imperialism: The Biological Expansion of Europe 900–1900* (London: Canto, 1986).

early nineteenth century, British colonization of India and the subsequent political, social, economic and ecological changes brought about led to the disease becoming, first, endemic throughout the region and then pandemic, affecting millions of people around the world. In his critical history of imperialism and disease, Watts (1997) describes how the building of irrigation canals without proper drainage to raise cash crops and the building of the continental railway were accompanied by the displacement and impoverishment of people by British land reforms. Consequently, cholera spread from India in 1817 in the first of six pandemics over the next hundred years. Upon reaching Europe, cholera found fertile ground to spread widely and repeatedly in epidemic proportions, becoming a much feared killer among the urban poor (Lee and Dodgson 2000).

A similar story is found with tuberculosis (TB), responsible for one in ten deaths in Europe during the nineteenth century (Jamison et al. 1993). TB was responsible for about a quarter of deaths in the US and England in the mid nineteenth century, and the chief cause of death in the US until 1909 (Spink 1978: 219). TB has long been associated with conditions of socioeconomic inequality, thriving in crowded, damp and unsanitary living conditions. As Porter and Ogden (1998) describe,

> In the late eighteenth century, the onset of the Industrial Revolution and the decline of agricultural employment together created the conditions for large-scale migration into the cities … the majority of the population were living in appalling, overcrowded conditions and that areas with the greatest poverty suffered the highest mortality rates. The overcrowded conditions in the urban slums undoubtedly contributed to the transmission of infection. It was recognized in 1899 that 'the most powerful factors in producing tuberculosis are: (a) air contaminated by the so called tubercle bacillus; (b) food inadequate in purity, quality, quantity, (c) confined and overcrowded dwellings; (d) a low state of general health and resisting power of the body.

Another major killer was influenza. Detailed analysis of past influenza pandemics is hindered by the lack of accurate historical data, the rapidly changing nature of the infectious agent, and the seasonality of the disease. Despite these challenges, medical historians identify periodic pandemics occurring over millennia of varying lethality depending on the particular strain. Interestingly, influenza remains one of the most 'global' of diseases because of its 'democratic' nature – the disease infects individuals without discrimination by socioeconomic class, sex or age (although mortality is usually higher among the very young and the elderly). Nonetheless, crowded living conditions increase the risk of infection, and poor diet and general health increase the vulnerability to secondary infections such as pneumonia. Thus, case fatality is higher among poorer social groups (Katz 1974: 417). Furthermore, the spread of influenza was closely related to prevailing modes of transport. As Patterson (1996) writes, 'At no time did the rate of spread exceed the speed of human travel, which for most of the period was by foot, horse, or sail. Influenza was, of course, spread much more rapidly in 1889 than ever before, through railroad and steamship travel. The pandemics of 1791 and 1830 moved at a more leisurely pace than the others.' Or as Walters (1978: 857) puts it, influenza 'spread in Turkistan with the speed of a caravan, in Europe of an express train, and over seas with the rapidity of ocean travel'.

This is most dramatically illustrated by the worst influenza pandemic in history (1918–19) which killed an estimated 20–40 million people (see Box 2.3). The mobility of military personnel, refugees and others following the First World War was a major factor in the spread of the disease to civilian populations across national borders, along with the disruption of public health systems during the war. Patterns of migration and urbanization may also have contributed to the pandemic. At the turn of the century, immigrants from Italy, Russia, Austria, Poland and French Canada migrated from rural villages to many US cities especially in the northeast (Walters 1978: 857). It is believed that many of these immigrants were especially susceptible because they had not been previously exposed to the influenza virus. Immigrants were aged between 14 and 44 years, three-quarters were male, and most were seeking employment as unskilled industrial labourers. Without the opportunity to develop immunity, they were ideal victims for the 1918–19 pandemic. Hence, these ethnic groups suffered higher rates of mortality from influenza than earlier immigrants (such as the Irish, English and Germans) (Katz 1974; 1977). A discussion of the contemporary risks of a comparably lethal influenza pandemic amid recent forms of globalization is discussed in Chapter 3.

The significant rise in urban mortality rates during the early period of European industrialization (early nineteenth century), marked by sharp differentials in rates of mortality and life expectancy between social groups,[2] prompted growing concern in Europe for social reform. An important aspect of the resultant efforts to improve public health domestically was the need to give increased attention to the determinants of health that lay abroad. The permeability of national borders to diseases was widely acknowledged given the experiences of cholera, TB and other infectious diseases described above. In addition, periodic outbreaks of vector-borne diseases demonstrated the need to understand so-called tropical diseases. Perhaps the most notable was the outbreak of yellow fever in Britain in 1865, transported by a cargo ship bringing iron ore from Cuba to Swansea (Desowitz 1997: 217–19). Wars during the twentieth century led to an increase in malaria. The First World War (1914–18) and the Russian Revolution (1919) brought *Plasmodium falciparum* as far north as Archangel. The Spanish Civil War, with its intervention by troops from Morocco, followed by the Second World War in 1939, brought an increase in malaria amid disrupted administration of drugs; the disease was finally eradicated in 1962 (de Zulueta 1994: 12). In reality, of course, the spread of tropical diseases was most pronounced among the tropical regions of the world as a result of increased trade and other links. For example, the spread

---

Box 2.3   The global influenza pandemic of 1918–19

Influenza remains one of the oldest and most common diseases known. Hippocrates records an epidemic in 412 BC and since then 31 possible influenza pandemics have been documented. Influenza is an acute respiratory illness caused by influenza viruses A and B. It is a disease that comes in seasonal epidemics and its occurrence is due to minor changes in the viral antigenic proteins (antigenic drift). Occasionally a major change to the virus occurs (antigenic shift) resulting in worldwide epidemics (pandemics). When this occurs, the 'new' form of the virus can affect large portions of the population and cause higher than usual morbidity and mortality.

The worst known influenza pandemic in history occurred at the end of the First World War (1918–19) resulting in up to 700 million cases worldwide and 20–40 million deaths (compared with 4.9 million war-related deaths during the war). The pandemic affected virtually all parts of the world over a short period of time. It occurred in three waves: (a) spring of 1917 to spring 1918; (b) September 1918 for about six to eight weeks; and (c) spring 1919. The second wave had by far the greatest impact (Gernhart 1999), killing at least 2% of a population each month, although figures vary given the likelihood of under-reporting and inaccurate diagnosis. This conservative figure is comparable to the impact of the plague epidemic in London during the fifteenth century (Weinstein 1976). In the US, one in four people contracted the virus, and there were between 500,000 and 1.5 million deaths. In India, six months of influenza led to almost as many deaths as caused by cholera in twenty years (Walters 1978: 855–56).

As well as high mortality, the pandemic had an unusual mortality distribution. Unlike previous strains, the virus affected 20–40-year-olds in particular, a feature still not explained by epidemiologists. There was also a puzzling pattern of spread, with the disease appearing almost simultaneously in distant locations such as New York and Bombay, yet taking days and even weeks to travel far shorter distances (New York to Chicago). Nor is it understood why Spain was the location for the index case (hence the name Spanish flu). The origins of the virus remain the subject of intense research. The infectious agent continued to elude scientists until 1933 when the human influenza virus was finally isolated, creating hopes that it could then be vanquished with emerging scientific weapons. There is some evidence that the virus was transported by southern Chinese labourers living in Europe and building many of the trenches of the First World War (Shortridge 1999). Chinese economic migration has occurred over many centuries, contributing significantly, for example, to the building of the railways in North America. It is known today that southern China serves as an influenza epicentre for new strains because of the close proximity of human and animal populations. It remains unknown, however, whether the 1918 pandemic was initially present in pigs before transmission to humans, or whether the virus found a reservoir in pigs after the pandemic. Recent gene sequencing research on lung tissue preserved from three victims of the 1918 pandemic suggests that the origins of the virus, in both its human and swine forms, may even be avian. The virus may have developed around 1905 and been introduced into the human population thereafter.

of schistosomiasis throughout Asia, Africa and Latin America occurred through the movement of workers between major irrigation systems. Similar factors led to the spread of dengue fever to the islands of the Pacific and parts of Asia (Cohen 1989: 53).

While concern for the health impacts on local people and migrant workers may have been a consideration, the risks posed by tropical diseases to Europeans seeking to extend their political and economic reach were the primary impetus behind the growth in scientific and public health attention to such diseases. Colonial and commercial interests, led by the British, supported the establishment of specialist training and research institutions such as the Liverpool School of Tropical Medicine (1898) and London School of Hygiene and Tropical Medicine (1899). The former was largely funded by commercial interests which enjoyed a lucrative trade with West Africa. Sir Alfred Jones, chairman of the Elder Dempster Line, the major passenger shipping line to the region, was the driving force behind the founding of the school (Desowitz 1997: 145). Other European countries followed suit with similar institutions, including the Karolinska Institute in Amsterdam, Holland, Prince Leopold Institute of Tropical Medicine in Antwerp, Belgium (1906), and Swiss Tropical Institute in Basel, Switzerland (1943).

In the US, the Rockefeller International Health Board (later the Rockefeller Foundation) was founded in 1913 by John D. Rockefeller, the industrialist who built his fortune through the Standard Oil Company. His early philanthropic efforts, in addition to contributing to the building of schools of tropical medicine in North America and Europe, centred on the eradication of hookworm. These efforts were initially focused on the American South, but eventually became international beginning in countries dominated by US commercial interests such as Panama, Costa Rica, Colombia and Nicaragua. In all of these countries, the productivity of the labour force of the United Fruit Company suffered from the disease (Farley 1995; Birn and Solarzano 1999). Yellow fever was also a major target of early programmes. Regardless of motives, the late nineteenth century onwards was a period of significant discovery in tropical diseases including the mosquito transmission of malaria, yellow fever and filariasis; tsetse fly transmission of African sleeping sickness; and snail transmission of schistosomiasis.

Internationally, governments recognized that any efforts to moderate the threats posed to economic interests by health risks required some degree of cooperation. While a limited degree of bilateral and regional cooperation had already been organized,[3] the first International Sanitary Conference held in 1851 marks the beginning of what Fidler (2001) calls 'international health diplomacy'. Over the next six decades, twelve international sanitary conferences were held to discuss matters of joint concern, notably the control of selected infectious disease. Of foremost importance was the need to minimize their adverse impacts on burgeoning trade links, a priority that defined the forms of cooperation agreed. There was strong support among many conference attendees for improving information on diseases such as yellow fever, cholera and plague, and equally strong rejection of attention to broader health issues, notably the social conditions that contribute to poor health. A total of four conventions were eventually agreed which were codified and consolidated into the International Sanitary Conventions of 1903. In addition, the same meeting agreed on the creation of a permanent organization for maintaining and reporting epidemiological data, and coordinating quarantine measures. Hence, the Office International d'Hygiène de Publique (OIHP) was established in Paris in 1907.

It was this early form of 'enlightened self-interest' that strongly defined international health cooperation until the end of the First World War. Powerful vested interests sought to protect and extend their political and economic reach through specific measures that protected trade and commerce. In contrast, there was growing support for greater attention to 'social medicine' led by charitable organizations such as the League of Red Cross Societies and the Save the Children Fund (both founded in 1919). A rethinking of international health cooperation was to be prompted by the horrors of the First World War and its aftermath.

2.5 The rise of international health (1920s to 1950s)

As in such fields as transportation, communication and education, there was a desire to develop greater international health cooperation following the end of the First World War as a means of fostering the spirit of international community. As Weindling (1995: 2) writes, the interwar period is characterized by 'the transition from treaties and conventions between nation states to the establishment of a brave new world of international organisations, designed to promote health and welfare'. During the 1920s, many governmental and nongovernmental organizations (NGOs) supported a vision of international health governance defined by humanitarianism. Many medical practitioners and public health officials building national health systems during this time became involved in international health, bringing with them a strong belief that concerted efforts needed to be directed at providing health care to all people. The principle of universality began to be increasingly popular in terms of access by all people to basic health care, as well as the inclusion of all countries in a system of international health cooperation (Dodgson et al. 2002).

These hopes were pinned on the Health Organization of the League of Nations, founded in 1920 and envisioned to play a more active role in fostering efforts to prevent the resurgence of diseases such as typhus and influenza, and not simply collecting data on their incidence. Yet almost immediately, high-level diplomatic tensions between internationalism and isolationism, marked by the decision of the US not to be a member of the League of Nations, impacted directly on the authority of the new organization. In addition, ongoing institutional rivalry between the new health organization and the OIHP prevented them from working more closely together throughout the interwar period (Dubin 1995). In some ways, the disparate nature of international health cooperation until the end of the Second World War was a reflection of the state of health services at the national level. Berridge describes the UK, for example, and the 'chaotic and uncoordinated nature of health services in terms of distribution, access, financing and much else' (Berridge 1999: 10). In the US the Communicable Disease Center (CDC), forerunner of the Centers for Disease Control, was established in 1946 with a mission to work with state and local health officials to control malaria and other communicable diseases. In general, governments were struggling with the challenge of building health systems that would effectively meet the needs of it domestic populations.

There were more successful efforts at building international health governance at the regional level. In 1902 governments in the Americas established the International Sanitary Bureau of the Americas, renamed the Pan American Sanitary Bureau (PASB) in 1923, and the forerunner of the Pan American Health Organization (PAHO). As the world's first permanent international health organization, the PASB played an important role in collecting epidemiological data and exchanging information with other organizations. Unlike other bodies, however, the PASB also played an active operational role, for example, initiating a campaign to eradicate yellow fever in the region. Its work was supported by the active role of charitable foundations, notably the Rockefeller Foundation, in the region.

The hard-won lessons of the Second World War brought a significant expansion in international health cooperation through the establishment of new institutions and official development assistance (ODA) for health purposes. Within the UN system, the World Health Organization (WHO) was created in 1948 as the UN specialized agency for health.[4] WHO was similar in many ways to the Health Organization of the League of Nations in that the ideal of universality forms the core of its mandate. Even in the face of scepticism at the attainability of such a goal, and continued ideological opposition to 'social medicine', WHO was and remains committed to an inclusive and rights-based vision of health for all. The establishment of six regional offices, and the decentralized nature of their resources and operations, embodied the aspiration to be a health organization for the world. It is notable that WHO is also strongly defined by its focus on intergovernmental cooperation, more specifically, the ministries of health of its member states. While NGOs could enter into official relations with the organization, in practice, they played a limited role until the 1970s.

Bilateral aid to the developing world by the governments of industrialized countries was also established during this period. For the US and its allies, development aid was an extension of foreign policy and an instrument in waging the Cold War. Hence, policies focused on building infrastructure, such as transport, or providing military aid. The scope of health sector aid was therefore narrowly circumscribed, with a strong emphasis on infectious disease control.

While the UN and bilateral aid agencies became the focus of international health cooperation among governments,[5] NGOs were also becoming more prominent. Church missions had been well-established providers of health services in Africa, Asia and Latin America since the nineteenth century, often acting as the sole source of health care. Newer nonstate actors focused on specific causes, such as emergency relief, human rights, women and children, or refugees, or on particular countries, notably the developing world. International NGOs, such as the Save the Children Fund and League of Red Cross Societies, formed local branches in many countries to facilitate their work. Others, such as Christian Aid, focused on coordinating aid centrally and then sending expertise, medicines and other resources to communities in need. Still others formed during emergency situations and then disbanded. All of these types of activities foreshadowed the explosion of NGO activity in the health sector from the 1970s.

2.6   Conclusion

There is a thought-provoking display at the Dinosaur Museum in Dorchester in the UK that speculates about what dinosaurs might have looked like had they not suffered mass extinction 65 million years ago. The hypothetical creature is remarkably humanoid suggesting that such a form is of some inherent evolutionary value. Yet the display also tells us about the sheer luck of *Homo sapiens* who, if it were not for a freak accident, would not have had the evolutionary space to eventually dominate the earth. As well as raising the question of whether dinosaurs would have made a better job of being the earth's caretaker, the exhibit drew appropriate attention to the fragility of evolutionary trajectories.

Patterns of health and disease have always been key factors in shaping those trajectories, from earliest human history to the present day. The direction is neither linear nor progressive, but fraught with shifting forces that challenge our intellectual capacities to make collective sense of them. Sources of food and water, social structures, cultural practices, communication patterns, conflict, local flora and fauna, and natural disasters have all played a direct role in how healthy or unhealthy societies have been. Conversely, the health of populations has been highly influential in the course of history. Human societies and health have been constantly intertwined.

It is thus important to begin with an historical timescale that acknowledges the multiplicity of factors that have shaped patterns of health and disease over time. From small bands of hunter-gatherers, to the large and highly urbanized megacities that we have today, the gradual changes brought about are an integral part of the history of human health. In terms of the conceptual framework of this book, the initial impact of globalization on health can be seen as largely spatial, as *Homo sapiens* migrated outwards from Africa to extend the territorial range of human societies. As communities settled and grew, the density of populations and their interactions with one another influenced the timescale in which changes to health occurred. Most prominently, the rate at which infectious diseases could spread was increased because of more densely populated communities. As human interaction intensified further, knowledge and ideas about health were communicated across communities.

It is in this context that the current phase of globalization, from the 1970s onwards, can be understood. On the one hand, the patterns of health and disease we can observe today are inextricably linked with social and natural history. On the other hand, however, there are distinct features of globalization from the late twentieth century that are having particular impacts on human health. To the extent that there are simultaneously spatial, temporal and cognitive dimensions of globalization at play, and that these changes are occurring with unprecedented intensity, it can be argued that this stage of globalization is distinct. There is accumulating evidence that the health impacts are also unique. During the twentieth century, there have been historic strides in health status reflecting improvements in social and physical living conditions. For hundreds of years, life expectancy at birth remained around 25–30 years. In 1900 average life expectancy in the US was 47 years, with only 3 per cent of the population over the age of 65 years (Moyer 2000). By the mid 1990s, this figure had increased to 70 years on average worldwide, and as much as 78 years for men and 82 years for women in some high-income countries (WHO 1996b).

The undoubted achievements in health status, when considered from a global perspective, are less impressive. Marked inequalities in health define contemporary forms of globalization. In the poorest countries life expectancy is 43 years while infant mortality rates (death of children under the age of one) vary from 4.8 per 1000 live births in high-income countries, to 161 per 1000 live births in low-income countries (WHO 1995). Nor are the health challenges confined to the developing world. Unprecedented growth of human populations is occurring at rates that pose a serious threat to the carrying capacity of the earth, worsened by the unsustainable lifestyles of the well-off. The spectre of emerging and re-emerging diseases is now widely recognized as a direct threat to the health gains of the past. The spread of antimicrobial-resistant 'superbugs' throughout the world raises serious doubts about our strong reliance in the past on scientific weapons to protect us. The world is bracing itself for a global pandemic of tobacco-related diseases in twenty years' time, as today's smokers begin to suffer the health consequences of their habit. So there is a plethora of both new and familiar health challenges that face us. It is the premise of this book that globalization processes are a core component of the ongoing story of human health, and that how effectively we tackle these emerging health issues will have direct consequences for the long-term sustainability of a global world order.

Key Readings

G. Berlinguer (1992), 'The Interchange of Disease and Health between the Old and New Worlds', *American Journal of Public Health*, October, 82(10): 1407–13.

Mark Nathan Cohen (1989), *Health and the Rise of Civilization* (New Haven: Yale University Press).

Alfred W. Crosby (1972), *The Columbian Exchange, Biological and Cultural Consequences of 1492* (Westport, Conn.: Greenwood Press, 1972).

Tony McMichael (2001), *Human Frontiers, Environments and Disease, Past Patterns, Uncertain Futures* (Cambridge: Cambridge University Press).

William McNeill (1976), *Plagues and People* (New York: Anchor Press/Doubleday).

3
The Spatial Dimension of Global Health

Our world has never been compartmentalized.
Robert Desowitz, *Who gave Pinta to the Santa Maria?* (1997)

3.1 Introduction

The spatial dimension of global change is perhaps the most readily acknowledged aspect of globalization through its redefining of the geographical boundaries that circumscribe our interactions with one another. The now somewhat clichéd vision of the 'global village' juxtaposes the local and the faraway, a world increasingly 'a single place' (Scholte 1997b) brought together by commonalities of experience, lifestyle, values and aspirations. But more than this, the global village implies a shared fate from forces that readily cross territorial space to affect all of our lives – transborder flows of people, goods and services, knowledge and ideas, environmental change and so on. Globalization is thus about changes to how we perceive and experience physical space, both individually and collectively.

As described in Chapter 2, the history of the human species is an ongoing evolutionary process of adaptation and change. From the prehistoric spread of the *Homo* genus from Africa into Europe and Asia, to the crossing of land bridges to the Americas and Australia, the human species has long been on the move. In the search for food and other resources, new territories were explored and increasingly sophisticated systems of delineating possession of such territories developed. As communities gradually grew larger and more permanent, the world was demarcated into defined territorial spaces – tribal lands, kingdoms, empires and more recently, sovereign states. Precise physical boundaries have been continually redrawn over time as a result of cooperation and conflict, but a specific location in a given territorial space has remained a core defining feature of human societies to the present day.

Are the changes that we are experiencing today, as a result of globalization, simply a continuation of this historical process of territorial delineation? Or are there distinct impacts on how we define social space and interact within it? More specifically, given the focus of this book, what implications do such changes have for human health? The link between the spatial dimension of global change and human health is twofold. First, the structure of human societies is changing in terms of territorial size, location and patterns of interaction, including the emergence of communities that are independent of territorial space. These spatial changes, in turn, are having significant impacts on geographical patterns of health and disease. Second, this changing geography of human health is, in turn, shaping the direction and nature of globalization as it is unfolding at the present time. Emerging global patterns of health and disease have important implications for the long-term sustainability of a globalized world order.

This chapter examines this mutual relationship as part of the spatial dimension of globalization and health. It begins by defining how globalization is leading to new concepts of geography. This is illustrated through three key manifestations of spatial change – the emerging global economy, global environmental change and global demographic trends. Each of these is explored in relation to its impacts on human health. The chapter concludes that a reterritorialization of health is under way that we are only beginning to understand and address.

3.2   Globalization as a new geography

Empire establishes no territorial center of power and does not rely on fixed boundaries and barriers. It is a decentered and deterritorializing apparatus of rule that progressively incorporates the entire global realm within its open, expanding frontiers.

Michael Hardt and Antonio Negri, *Empire* (2000)

The spatial dimension of global change concerns the ways in which physical or territorial space is being altered by globalizing forces. The defining principle for territorially dividing the world today is the sovereign state. The modern states system, of course, is a relatively recent organizing principle. While states existed before the Thirty Years War

(1618–48), the treaties signed in 1648 by warring European powers to end hostilities created the legal and political framework of modern interstate relations. Known as the Peace of Westphalia, the treaties established a number of important principles – recognition of a society of states based on the principle of territorial sovereignty; the independence of states with jural rights that other states are bound to respect; the legitimacy of different forms of government; and the notion of religious freedom and tolerance. In doing so, the medieval notion of a universal religious authority acting as final arbiter of Christendom was abolished and replaced by notions such as 'reason of state' and 'balance of power'. The Westphalian states system, of course, was primarily Christian and European, and would not embrace other parts of the world until the nineteenth and twentieth centuries (Evans and Newnham 1992: 343).

While the states system endures today as the core organizing principle of world politics, it is widely held that globalization is eroding the relative importance of the state. A minimalist perspective on globalization argues that there has been a quantitative increase in human activity across state-defined borders. As a result, the importance of what happens within state boundaries is being increasingly influenced by what happens across state boundaries. Crossborder exchanges have long been an important feature of the modern states system. It is argued that what is distinct today is the volume of such exchanges in the form, for example, of international trade of goods and services, documented migrants,[1] and foreign aid and investment.

It remains contested whether increased interstate or international exchanges reinforce or undermine the state. Strictly speaking, Scholte (1997: 15) defines such 'a process of intensifying connections between national domains' as *internationalization* rather than *globalization*. Crossborder flows bring people closer together through greater interaction across national borders, but the importance of the state as a territorially defined entity remains of key importance in regulating such exchanges in the form of trade agreements, customs inspections and immigration policies. A stricter use of the term globalization seeks to find qualitative differences in how we perceive and experience physical space. As Scholte (2000: 46–50) explains, our sense of place has traditionally referred to a location on a map, with the earth divided in varying ways (for example cities, districts, counties, provinces, states, countries and regions). Our measures of location and distance are tied to latitude, longitude and altitude. With globalization, new forms of social space are emerging that are not entirely territorial (cyberspace and the Internet; network society), thus reconfiguring social space towards transborder or non-territorial relations. It is this 'deterritorialization' or 'supraterritorialization' of human interaction that is a core feature of globalization.

Scholte (2000: 55) identifies a range of global activities that are detached, to varying degrees, from territorial logic – communications (telephone calls, satellite television), markets (global products and sales strategies), production (global production chains), money, finance, social ecology and consciousness. Some of these emerging forms of social space may reinforce the importance of the state, perhaps requiring collective action by many states, while others directly contradict and undermine territorial state sovereignty. Scholte writes that '[g]lobalization is not dissolving the state, but it has not left it untouched either. The challenge ... is to determine how the growth of supraterritorial social space is altering the activities and role of the state in contemporary history' (Scholte 1997: 22).

Overall, the rise of new forms of social space challenges us to adjust our traditional approaches to understanding determinants of health. How we define the health needs of human populations remains strongly premised on conventional notions of territory. Public health is not as fixated on the state as the study of international relations, but does rely to a large extent on notions of population groups located in territorially fixed spaces. Health systems, in turn, are historically constructed along national lines. The quantitative growth in crossborder exchanges requires us to recognize the permeability of certain territorial boundaries, leading to a reterritorialization of populations and the physical spaces within which they live and interact. The growth of transborder exchanges is a qualitative change that introduces the notion of deterritorialized social space. Both types of change are considered below in relation to their potential impacts on human health.

3.3   The health implications of an emerging global economy

> *Even though the world is incomparably richer than ever before, ours is also a world of extraordinary deprivation and of staggering inequality.*
>
> Amartya Sen (2001)

One of the key global changes affecting the organization of social space concerns the restructuring of economic relations. The emerging global economy is often cited as the key driver of globalization, bringing about changes in other spheres of social interaction through new forms of production, exchange (trade) and consumption. Scholte (2000: 430) usefully differentiates the changes taking place along three lines: (a) crossing of borders; (b) opening of borders; and (c) transcendence of borders. The first, as described above, is defined as *internationalization*. In spatial terms, economic entities located in separate politically defined territories engage in the exchange of goods and services. This may be between city-states, great empires or, since the establishment of the states system in the fifteenth century, sovereign states. Analyses of economic globalization using this definition have invited some scepticism whether there is much quantitatively, and certainly qualitatively, new actually happening (Hirst and Thompson 1995).

The second distinction, the opening of borders, concerns the *liberalization* of flows of economic inputs and outputs, and production processes, from nationally imposed restrictions. Since 1945 there has been a succession of regional and international agreements, based largely around the General Agreement on Tariffs and Trade (GATT) and its successor the World Trade Organization (WTO), that seek to reduce or remove restrictions on trade. The types of economic activity subsumed under trade agreements have steadily grown, with prospects in future negotiations of encompassing foreign direct investment (FDI), services and the agricultural sector. In spatial terms, the opening of borders through trade liberalization has encouraged economic entities located in different countries to pursue markets further afield. This has led to a further growth in international trade dominated by larger and larger concerns led by transnational corporations (TNCs). Of the largest one hundred economic entities in the world today, countries comprise fifty while the remainder are private companies. In the mid 1990s, 350 of the largest corporations accounted for 40 per cent of international trade (UNDP 1997).

The third category of change is the most radical in terms of altering the spatial dimension of economic relations. As Scholte (2000: 434) writes, *globalization* refers to 'processes whereby social relations acquire relatively distanceless and borderless qualities, so that human lives are increasingly played out in the world as a single place. In this usage, "globalization" refers to a fundamental transformation of geography ... [author's emphasis]'. In such an economy, patterns of production, exchange and consumption are increasingly delinked from territorial space, instead extending across widely dispersed locations to transcend national borders. It is this increase in transborder or supraterritorial activities that Dicken (1998: 2) describes as the 'global shift' towards 'a new geo-economy' whereby

> The straightforward exchange between core and periphery areas, based upon a broad division of labour, is being transformed into a highly complex, kaleidoscope structure involving the fragmentation of many production processes and their geographical relocation on a global scale in ways which slice through national boundaries.

The increased complexity of the corporate world, with huge conglomerates owning a diverse range of companies through vertical and horizontal integration of industries, reflects this globalizing trend. As an indicator of the accelerated pace and scope of corporate restructuring, crossborder mergers and acquisitions rose from US$0.9 trillion worldwide in 1996 to US$3.4 trillion in 1999 (Corrigan 1999). As Mooney (1999: 76) states: 'We are talking about sudden and enormous concentrations of power.'

An intensifying and increasingly liberalized international economy, and an emerging global economy, poses potentially varied impacts on human health. These are considered below in relation to three major health-related industries – pharmaceuticals, food and tobacco. Before doing so, it is useful to review the main concerns being raised regarding the changing nature of the world economy and its health consequences. The first is the argument that the emerging global economy is contributing to worsening inequalities within and across countries. This is impoverishing a substantial proportion of humanity and, in turn, adversely affecting their health status. There is substantial evidence of increasing socioeconomic inequality within and across countries in recent decades. Using a variety of measures, such as purchasing power parity (PPP), Gini coefficient and world economic distribution, most economic analyses demonstrate that the number of poor people, and the income gap between the rich and the poor, has increased. While at least one-fifth of the world's population lives in absolute poverty (less than US$1 per day), the richest 225 people in the world have a combined wealth of US$1 trillion (equal to the annual income of the poorest 47 per cent of the world's population of 2.5 billion people) (UNDP 1997). Put another way, 20 per cent of people in high-income countries account for 86 per cent of private consumption while the poorest 28 per cent consume 1.3 per cent (Navarro 1999a: 219).

What remains in hot dispute are the causes of these inequalities. Neoliberal theory, the dominant view since the 1980s, argues that competitive markets yield the greatest economic growth which, in turn, eventually leads to a 'trickling down' of benefits to other social classes including the poor. Although there may be an initial widening of the gap between rich and poor with the generation of wealth by the relatively well off, their use of this wealth to create employment, buy goods and services, and invest gradually enables others in society to share in the economic benefits. If this fails to happen, neoliberals argue that this is due to the failure by some governments to sufficiently embrace appropriate economic reforms, hence not allowing market forces to work their magic (Dollar and Kraay 2000). After many decades of neoliberal-based reforms, and with the mixed experiences of highly varied economies to learn from, most analysts now temper their ardour for solely market-led solutions. There is recognition that winners and losers are created along the way to economic growth, and that appropriate public policies are needed to cushion the negative impacts felt by some during the transition period (Wade 2001; Cornea 2001). Further discussion of how neoliberal ideas have underpinned health sector reforms since the 1980s is provided in Chapter 5.

In contrast, critics of neoliberalism strongly dispute its core assumptions. One major criticism is that there is something inherently unfair about current forms of global capitalism which, like a 'stacked' deck of cards, invariably leads to enduring inequalities. Unequal ownership or access to the means of production and exchange, for example, means that certain social classes are unable to participate fairly, and share in the benefits, of much economic activity. Existing terms of trade mean that producers of primary products, raw materials and natural resources may receive a disproportionately small share of earnings. Unfair protectionist practices mean that some high-income countries push for the opening of markets for their own exports, but maintain barriers against the imports of other countries, notably in the agricultural sector. Intellectual property laws upheld by the World Trade Organization (WTO) and World Intellectual Property Organization (WIPO) allow large corporations to exert ownership of, and hence the right to reap profits from, valuable resources found in the developing world (for example local flora) or that should arguably remain in the public domain. Most blameworthy of all, perhaps, it is argued that a small number of countries have defined the structure and operating rules of the world economy in such a way as to advantage their interests. The continued exclusivity of key multilateral economic institutions such as the WTO, World Bank, International Monetary Fund (IMF) and Organization for Economic Cooperation and Development

(OECD) attests to the inability of other interests to challenge the system.

In an international economy, the inequalities manifest between rich and poor countries. Within the emerging global economy, means of production are seen as controlled by a transnational elite operating within and across countries, pursuing wealth creation across the world without regard to territorial space. Among this elite are large TNCs that are able to control the most valuable natural and human resources, the largest sources of capital and investment, and the core technologies and know-how (Korten 2001). Furthermore, this 'transnational managerial class' is highly mobile, able to move capital, investment, production facilities and other operations to those parts of the world that provide optimal return. This creates leverage over individuals and groups – national governments, unskilled workers – that are relatively fixed territorially. Hence, as many major industries have undergone restructuring over recent decades, to adjust to an increasingly global marketplace, losers have been created through the 'downsizing' of work forces, downward pressures on wages, and displacement of smaller local producers (Navarro 1998; Schuftan 1999).

It would be overly simplistic, however, merely to equate globalization with rampant capitalism. It would also be incomplete to limit globalization, with all of its inherent contradictions, to a north–south battlefield. Rather, it is argued here that a new geography of winners and losers are being created, admittedly emerging from pre-existent patterns of wealth creation and distribution, but distinct too in the new forms of social organization being formed. The global economy, that Hardt and Negri (2000) call the 'Empire', has no territorial boundaries, being both nowhere and everywhere:

> The spatial divisions of the three Worlds (First, Second and Third) have been scrambled so that we continually find the First world in the Third, the Third world in the First, and the Second almost nowhere at all. Capital seems to be faced with a smooth world – or really, a world defined by new and complex regimes of differentiation and homogenization, deterritorialization and reterritorialization.

The health implications of inequality are well documented. The most direct link is that poor people have greater difficulty meeting those basic needs that contribute to good health. One-quarter of the world's population does not have access to safe drinking water, and one-third are inadequately sheltered and clothed. Fourteen million children die of hunger each year (Navarro 1999a: 218), while over twelve million children under the age of five years die annually from preventable diseases (Save the Children 1996). Eight hundred million people lack access to public health care and half the world's population lacks regular access to essential drugs. These are sobering statistics when contrasted with the relative abundance of the well-off.

Also important are relative inequalities. Evidence suggests that economic globalization is producing greater inequalities both within and across countries. As measured by the Human Poverty Index (HPI), one person in eight in high-income countries is affected by poverty – long-term unemployment, life expectancy of less than 60 years, income below the national poverty line or an inadequate level of literacy (UNDP 1999: 28). Wilkinson's (1996) seminal work demonstrates that relative poverty within a society creates adverse health impacts – what Farmer (2001: 5) calls the 'biological reflections of social fault lines'. From a global perspective, where there can be greater awareness of the differences between 'haves' and 'have nots' in other societies, unprecedented wealth for a relative few is having health consequences that cut across territorial boundaries.

A second feature of the emerging global economy is the vulnerability of local economies to events elsewhere as a result of greater interconnectedness. It is apt that the metaphor of 'contagion' has been adopted to describe the vulnerability of national economies to the economic problems of other countries within a global economic system (Chang and Majnoni 2000). The potentially greater volatility of local economic conditions, and the social consequences of this vulnerability, were demonstrated by the global financial crisis of the late 1990s. Data from East and Southeast Asia show that the financial crisis led to widespread unemployment and increased levels of poverty, as well as reduced access to health care and ultimately declines in health status among certain population groups. In Hong Kong, for example, the number of people living in poverty increased by 20 per cent between 1997 and 1999, accompanied by a sharp decline in private consumption of health services and increased utilization of public health services. In Indonesia, poverty levels increased by almost 80 per cent (comprising 20.3 per cent of the population). Similar findings from Thailand, South Korea, Malaysia, Singapore and Japan show reduced real per capita household income, real earnings per worker, rising unemployment and poverty levels (Chan 2001).

Third, health impacts arise from inappropriate or insufficient regulation of global economic activities that affect the determinants of

health. One of the main concerns expressed about economic globalization is the lagging behind of policies that protect and promote human
welfare. The *laissez faire* system that characterizes the emerging global
economy is a mish-mash of regulatory standards, partly national, to a
lesser extent international, and partly proto-global. The result is con-
siderable variation from country to country in the way economic entities are permitted to behave regarding, for example, occupational
health and safety standards, consumer safety, marketing, social welfare
provisions (such as unemployment, minimum wage) and environmental protection. For example, there is especially weak regulation in most
low-income countries of products with harmful health effects such as
tobacco, alcohol and food products. Similarly, spillover effects created
by certain externalities of global economic activity, such as pollution
and dumping of hazardous waste, has become a serious problem
because of the lack of congruence between national environmental
protection standards and the mobility of global business. To some
extent, this is due to a 'jurisdictional gap' (Kaul et al. 1999) in authority, with national governments lacking adequate capacity being unable
to hold large TNCs sufficiently accountable. At the same time many
governments are unwilling, and with structural adjustment programmes unable, to adopt taxation policies for improving social
welfare for fear of discouraging FDI.

Finally, there are potential *market failures* in the emerging global
economy that can lead to the underproduction of certain goods and
services desirable for the protection and promotion of health. For
example, by their nature, profit-seeking companies produce goods and
services that will bring them the greatest economic return. This is
unlikely to include the needs of the poorest within and across countries, those least able to pay for health care, yet those most likely to
need it. Similarly, so-called neglected diseases (see Chapter 5) are those
that too few suffer from, or again are too poor, to offer a profitable
return to companies to invest resources to develop interventions. This
can also lead to cream-skimming which is the tendency for markets to
provide the most profitable goods and services, at the expense of less
profitable, but socially beneficial, goods and services. Government provision of both types allows cross-subsidizing of the latter, but allowing
companies to 'cream off' profits undermines this.

Another market failure is the provision of public goods. Public
goods have the properties of being nonrival in consumption and
nonexcludable. The classic example is a lighthouse whereby its additional use by another individual does not add to its cost nor preclude

others from using it. In public health, public goods include immunization, and systems of surveillance and monitoring of infectious diseases. The problem is that public goods encourage free riders, those who enjoy its benefits without contributing to its cost. It is this free-rider problem that lies behind the concept of global public goods defined as

> a public good with benefits that are strongly universal in terms of countries (covering more than one group of countries), people (accruing to several, preferably all, population groups) and generations (extending to both current and future generations, or at least meeting the needs of current generations without foreclosing development options for future generations) (Kaul et al. 1999: 510)

To explore these challenges further, we now turn to three health-related industries that, through their increasingly globalized nature, illustrate some of the health impacts described above.

3.3.1 The globalization of the pharmaceutical industry

The public's health in the global era is, thus, intimately connected to the health of the global pharmaceutical industry.

Lasagna (1997)

Pharmaceuticals can be categorized as (a) in-patent drugs; (b) out-of-patent, generic or multi-source drugs; and (c) over-the-counter (OTC) or proprietary drugs. The world market for the first two categories (known as ethical products) was about US$255 billion (1995), and US$30.4 billion (1992) for OTCs (Chetley 1995). Since the late 1980s, a significant restructuring of the pharmaceutical industry has occurred towards the formation of larger and fewer companies. These larger companies have increased the scale of their operations, and diversified the range of their products, through a growing number of mergers and acquisitions, joint ventures and strategic alliances. Between 1994 and 1997 such deals were worth an estimated US$80 billion. In the five years between 1996 and 2001 this figure rose to US$500 billion. In 1999 alone it is estimated that deals totalled US$400 billion, with another US$100 billion changing hands during the first half of 2000 including the merger of Glaxo Wellcome and SmithKline Beecham (US$160 billion), and Pfizer and Warner-Lambert (US$85 billion) (Farrelly 2001a; Mooney 1999:77).

Over the past twenty years, the leading companies have remained somewhat static although their specific position in the industry has frequently shifted. The ten largest pharmaceutical companies (Table 3.1) accounted for about 47 per cent of world sales in 2000 (Farrelly 2001a). Within therapeutics submarkets, there is even greater concentration with the top three products commonly accounting for 45–60 per cent of total sales (Casidio Tarabusi and Vickery 1999a: 89). The pharmaceutical industry is also geographically dominated by companies based in a small number of countries, with companies based in OECD countries accounting for 92 per cent of exports, 78 per cent of imports and over 70 per cent of world production and consumption (Casidio Tarabusi and Vickery 1999a). Eighty per cent of the world's medicines are consumed by people in fifteen countries concentrated in the US, Europe and Japan (Pilling 1999a). In addition, the level of trade has increased significantly between 1980 and 1994, with total exports increasing from US$14 billion to US$57 billion. Indeed, trade has outpaced growth in production (US$75 to US$205 billion during the same period) in line with other manufacturing sectors, thus demonstrating a trend towards increased internationalization.

As well as greater concentration of ownership within a small number of companies and countries, Casidio Tarabusi and Vickery (1998) describe the industry as demonstrating a 'multi-country pattern of globalization'. This means that production, packaging and marketing has been extensively carried out in the countries of final sale, made necessary by the continued importance of national health regulations, the local incidence of particular diseases, and traditions of medical

Table 3.1   The world's top ten pharmaceutical companies

Company (headquarters)	Rank	Sales (US$billion)	Market share (%)
Pfizer (US)	1	23.1	7.3
GlaxoSmithKline (UK)	2	22.0	6.9
Merck (US)	3	16.5	5.2
Astra Zeneca (UK/Sweden)	4	14.3	4.5
Bristol-Myers Squibb (US)	5	13.3	4.2
Novartis (Switzerland)	6	12.4	3.9
Johnson & Johnson (US)	7	12.3	3.9
Aventis (Germany/France)	8	11.3	3.6
Pharmacia (Sweden/US)	9	10.2	3.2
American Home Products (US)	10	9.6	3.0

Source: As quoted in Farrelly P. (2001), 'Big ... and plotting to become bigger still', *The Observer*, 22 April: 3.

practice. This is especially notable in Asian countries, which are seen by the industry as the largest potential area of growth. The region presently represents less than 10 per cent of the world market. During the fifteen years up to the global financial crisis of 1997–98, market growth was exponential. With Asian populations expected to get older and richer, and to adopt Western diets and lifestyles (thus increasing the risk of so-called diseases of affluence), sales are expected to rise to 31 per cent of world sales by 2008 (Pilling 1999a).

Pressures on companies to remain competitive in the emerging market for pharmaceuticals have been the key drivers of industry globalization. One key area is research and development (R&D). The industry has long been among the top four most R&D intensive, with the highest spending companies allocating an average of 15 per cent of sales. Over the past two decades, R&D investment has doubled every five years from US$5.5 billion in 1981 to US$45 billion in 1996 (Walker 1997:66). It is estimated that the cost of developing a new drug is about US$300–400 million. Given the need for such substantial investment, economies of scale are critical to ensure an adequate volume of sales. The result has been the horizontal and vertical integration of the industry. For example, many large companies have joined with smaller biotechnology firms, through various alliances, licensing arrangements and shared ownership of companies, to develop new products. In other cases, rivals are bought out and integrated into increasingly global companies. As Casidio Tarabusi and Vickery (1999a: 88) write, 'The recent round of consolidation is global more than national, with firms acquiring rivals to gain global market share, rather than national shares. More firms with specialized portfolios of globally sold drugs are operating in all national markets.'

Another important development in the globalization of the pharmaceutical industry has been efforts to standardize intellectual property law protection across all countries. By 2005 low and middle-income countries are scheduled to adopt patent protection regimes in line with the Agreement on Trade-Related Intellectual Property Rights (TRIPS). The pharmaceutical industries in Thailand and India are particular targets of the agreement. India, for example, is the second largest pharmaceutical market in the world by volume but, because of low prices earned for generics and weak patent enforcement resulting in the pirating of new drugs, is thirteenth in value. India is estimated to have about 20,000 companies copying medicines developed elsewhere. The company Ranbaxy has production facilities in India and abroad, joint ventures in the US, China and Australia, and sales in thirty countries.

Box 3.1   A case study of GlaxoSmithKline

The origins of GlaxoSmithKline plc (GSK), one of the world's largest pharmaceutical companies, date from the eighteenth century. It was during the Industrial Revolution of the nineteenth century that many of the founders of the various companies that would eventually merge together to form GSK, established themselves – John K. Smith, Thomas Beecham, Mahlon Kline, Joseph Nathan, Henry Wellcome and Silas Burroughs. By the turn of the century, Smith, Kline & Company, Burroughs Wellcome & Company, Joseph Nathan & Company (the forerunner of Glaxo) and Beecham Pills Ltd. were all thriving concerns. Over the next fifty years or so, all the companies continued to expand their product lines through the development of new drugs, diversification and acquisition of other concerns. From the Second World War until the 1970s, these activities continued to grow as markets increased for prescription and over-the-counter (OTC) drugs in industrialized countries.

From the early 1980s, however, pressures to increase economies of scale and reach increasingly global markets led to a series of mergers and acquisitions as follows:

1982 SmithKline merges with Beckman Instruments to become SmithKline Beckman.

1989 SmithKline Beckman merges with The Beecham Group plc to become SmithKline Beecham plc.

1994 SmithKline Beecham acquires Diversified Pharmaceutical Services and Sterling Health to become third largest OTC medicines company.

1995 Glaxo and Burroughs Wellcome merge to form GlaxoWellcome.

1998 SmithKline Beecham plans to merge with American Home Products (AHP) but deal does not work out.

2000 GlaxoWellcome merges with SmithKline Beecham to form Glaxo-SmithKline in a US$160 billion deal.

2001 GlaxoSmithKline attempts merger with American Home Products in a deal worth US$225 billion to create the world's largest pharmaceuticals company but deal is ruled against by the UK Monopolies and Mergers Commission.

Today, GSK accounts for 7% of the world pharmaceutical market, with sales of US$27.5 billion (£18 billion) to 140 countries in 2000. The company leads in four therapeutic areas – anti-infectives (e.g. AZT for HIV/AIDS), central nervous system, respiratory (e.g. new asthma drug Advair) and gastric-intestinal/metabolic addition (e.g. ulcer treatment Zantac©).

The company is a good example of the shift, from national to international operations during the early to mid twentieth century, to an increasingly globalized structure and operations from the late twentieth century. It is ranked the 34th largest economic entity in the world, worth an estimated US$155 billion in 2001, with operating companies in 70 countries. In many ways, the company's activities maintain an international pattern of operation. Its headquarters remains the UK, with significant operations in the US, where control over key decision-making on corporate strategy and planning

Box 3.1 **continued**

remains. The US$4 billion (£2.5 billion) worth of R&D investment in 2000 activities also remains centralized in relatively few countries, with 16,000 employees located at 24 sites, principally in five countries (UK, US, Japan, Italy and Belgium).

At the same time, there are global aspects of the company's operations in terms of the decentralization of other activities such as the sourcing of inputs, manufacturing, sales and marketing. The company's 108 manufacturing sites, located in 41 countries, employ 39,000 people. Cheaper labour costs, along with national regulations, have required the company to establish manufacturing facilities in local markets. For example, the company built a US$130 million plant in Suzhou, China in 1999 to produce anti-infectives such as Lamivudine (Heptodin or Zeffix), the first oral treatment for Hepatitis B. The drug was developed and designed by BioChem Pharma of Canada and licensed to Glaxo in 1990, and largely intended for the Chinese market given 120 million carriers in China and 350 million worldwide (Pilling 1999a). In short, through horizontal and vertical integration, a core company has been formed but operates globally through a complex network of research laboratories, manufacturing plants bound together through licensing agreements, collaborative agreements, and joint ventures. While still constrained by national regulation, this diversity of operations increasingly blurs national boundaries.

Sources: James R. Rhodes, *Henry Wellcome* (London: Hodder & Stoughton 1994); Harding J., 'Case study Glaxo, Liver cure patently theirs', *Financial Times*, 15 July 1999, p. iv; P. Farrelly, 'Glaxo eyes £150 bn bid for US rival,' *Observer*, 22 April 2001, p. B1; and GSK (2001), *Annual Report 2000* (Greenford: GlaxoSmithKline).

Similarly, the Bombay-based company Ipca exports to more than sixty countries including Russia, North America and parts of Europe (Pilling 1999b).

As well as national compliance to TRIPS by 2005, there have been controversial attempts to enforce its provisions in selected countries in what Michael Bailey, Senior Policy Adviser to Oxfam, calls 'systematic intimidation' (as quoted in Boseley 2001a). A highly publicized example began in 1997 when 39 domestic and foreign pharmaceutical companies (including GlaxoSmithKline (GSK), Roche and Bristol-Myers Squibb) mounted a legal challenge to an amendment to the South African Medicines and Related Substances Control Amendment Act that would allow the import and use of cheaper generic versions of prescription medicines. The key clause, 15(c), states that South Africa can find and 'parallel import' the cheapest world price for a drug and impose 'compulsory drugs licensing' that grants rights to other companies to make copies of patented drugs. The main impetus for this amendment was the HIV/AIDS epidemic that had so far infected at least 16 per cent of the country's population. It is estimated that AIDS kills 5000 people a week. In 1999 the Minister of Health argued that budgetary constraints under the structural adjustment programme (SAP) prevented her from offering universal treatment to HIV-positive pregnant women, at a cost of US$13 million, that would save an estimated 30,000 lives. For example, Zidovudine (AZT), developed by the US National Institutes of Health (NIH) and produced under licence by GSK, costs US$240 per month in South Africa compared to an Indian-made generic at US$48 per month of treatment (Bond 1999). In April 2001, after much negative publicity, the pharmaceutical companies withdrew their legal action (McGreal 2001).

On the one hand, the case may bring greater access by the developing world to life-saving drugs. The legal action is seen by many as a public relations disaster for the industry, and many companies are keen to demonstrate their positive contribution to global health through corporate social responsibility policies, including cutting the price of selected drugs (Clark 2001b). The South African case may also affect the outcome of other efforts to enforce the TRIPS agreement. This includes a case lodged by the US government with the WTO in January 2001 against Article 68 of Brazil's Industrial Property Act 1996 which similarly allows the making or import of generic drugs for drugs not manufactured in the country. Brazil is seen as having a model treatment policy for HIV-positive patients by distributing anti-retroviral drugs to the majority of patients needing them. The Brazilian government has so far successfully negotiated with Merck to reduce the price of Efavirenz, one of two patented drugs costing one-third of the country's AIDS drugs budget (Boseley 2001a). The anthrax outbreaks following the terrorist attacks on the World Trade Center in September 2001 also dealt a blow to TRIPS by raising questions about the need to access generic drugs in a public health emergency (Singh 2002). A further undermining of the agreement came with the publication of the WHO list of approved drug companies which included a large Indian generic manufacturer and three smaller European companies. The list was seen as 'a setback for major multinational pharmaceutical companies, who want only patent-holders to be allowed to sell drugs and decide what discounts to offer' (McNeil 2002).

On the other hand, a number of concerns remain unresolved by the above events. Perhaps most immediately, there are fears that the market will be flooded with cheap and potentially dangerous or substandard drugs. More fundamental to the industry will be predictions of even greater concentration of ownership as companies jockey to meet the high costs of R&D and preserve their market share. Previous industry leaders, such as Bayer (Germany) and Roche (Switzerland), are expected to agree deals to put them back among the giants. Middle-ranking firms, such as Abbott, Eli Lilly and Schering Plough, may be the targets of such bids (Farrelly 2001b). The long-term implications for drug development (see Chapter 5) and pricing is unclear but a global industry with even larger and fewer companies will wield even greater influence over the health systems of the world.

3.3.2 The globalization of the food industry

> *It organizes the world from the perspective of satellite images (no political jurisdictions appear) ...*
>
> Kneen (1999) on the food company Cargill

Historically, human diets have evolved with the availability of new food sources, production and processing methods (Welch and Mitchell 2000), as well as knowledge about health and nutrition. In broad terms, there have been improvements in all of these areas, notably since the nineteenth century. While access to adequate amounts and quality of food, and levels of food security, remain highly variable across population groups, average daily caloric intake has increased worldwide alongside the capacity of the earth to produce sufficient food to feed ever larger populations. Two key features of food production and consumption patterns over the last several hundred years or so have been industrialization and globalization. Both raise questions about the long-term sustainability of food production, and the implications for patterns of health and disease.

In terms of food production, practices developed in Europe were gradually replicated in the New World and colonized territories alongside the development of capitalism. During the Industrial Revolution, the agricultural sector in Europe saw important shifts towards larger and fewer producers. These trends intensified during the twentieth century, facilitated by greater mechanization and technological advances. This rise of an 'agro-industrial complex' (McMichael 1998: 100) is characterized by both internationalization and globalization. The intensified internationalization of the food industry, by which food products of one country are exported to other countries under national, regional and international regulation, is evidenced by the greater scale of trade, and its farther geographical reach. Between 1980 and 2000, the proportion of imported fruit and vegetables consumed by Americans rose from 5.8 per cent and 5.9 per cent to 21.8 per cent and 14 per cent respectively. Seasonally, up to 70 per cent of selected fruit and vegetables consumed in the US comes from low-income countries (Wise 1997: 1641). Similarly, total food imports to Japan increased between 1985 and 2000 by about 200 per cent (from US$15.5 billion to US$46 billion) (Japan 2001).

The globalization of food production is where patterns of production have developed in ways that make territorial space less relevant. Lang (1998: 538) identifies a range of changes occurring in the food industry, some of them leading to increased internationalization, others to globalization:

- a rapid concentration of power in all sectors through mergers and acquisitions, or growth;
- fragmentation and volatility in consumer markets;
- rapid changes, driven by commercial interests, in diet and taste preferences;
- intensification of production;
- transformation of foods and food processes across all sectors;
- changes in the nature of farming, storage and consumption;
- a growth in the size and influence of food distributors and retailers;
- new inequalities within and between countries in food security;
- an ideological tension over the role of the state in regulation and education; and
- a battle for food markets between EU member states and the US (Lang 1999).

The model of agricultural production that we have today, one that is steadily being replicated worldwide, is characterized by mass production methods, capital (rather than labour) intensity, large economies of scale and 'bio-uniformity'.[2] McMichael (1998: 101) argues that the progression from multinational markets to transnational complexes is a result of changes in global capitalism from the 1970s leading to the relaxation of national controls on capital movements, the expansion of TNCs, and changes in US agricultural policy (for example the Farm Bill of 1973) to resolve balance of payments problems. The latter 'fundamentally altered the relation of American agriculture to the world economy', leading to a new dependency on foreign markets and intensified production methods. As in the pharmaceutical industry, vertical and horizontal integration of food producers has led to highly concentrated ownership in a smaller number of large companies during the late 1990s. Major deals include the purchase of the world's largest seed company, Pioneer Hi-Bred, by Dupont (US$7.7 billion), Monsanto's purchase of seed company stocks (about US$8.5 billion), and the acquisition of Monsanto itself by Pharmacia & Upjohn (US$37 billion). During the first half of 2000, a further US$150 billions-worth of acquisitions took place (Mooney 1999: 78). Box 3.2 presents a case study of Monsanto, one of the largest companies in the food production industry.

These trends have been further facilitated by efforts under multilateral trade agreements (MTAs) to liberalize the agricultural sector. Traditionally, the agricultural sector has been excluded from trade negotiations because of the reluctance by many countries to be too reliant on food imports. The protection of rural livelihoods has also been a sensitive political issue. The economic irrationality of some protectionist practices, such as the EU's Common Agricultural Policy (CAP), and the desire of large corporations to access new markets, have led to counter-pressures to include the agricultural sector in WTO trade negotiations. The extent to which the sector is liberalized as a result of these negotiations will have significant impacts on the emerging structure of the food production industry.

The health implications of a global food industry are many. First, there are concerns surrounding production processes themselves in terms of specific inputs, techniques and externalities. The intensification of production methods has, in large part, come from the increased use of certain chemicals in the form of fertilizers and pesticides, which may adversely affect health and/or the environment. Pesticide exports increased between 1961 and 1998 ninefold to US$11.4 billion per annum (French 2000). Public concern about pesticide residues has led to a thriving market for organic produce since the mid 1990s in many high-income countries. In the UK, the market for organic food increased from £30 million (US$45 million) in 1987 (Brown 2000) to more than £600 million (US$900 million) in 2001, including a 50% rise between 1999 and 2001 (Carslaw 2001). In the US, organic farming was one of the fastest growing segments of agriculture during the 1990s. USDA (2000) estimates that the annual value of retail sales of organic foods in 1999 was approximately US$6 billion, up from US$2.8 billion in 1996 (O'Neil 1996). The number of organic farmers is increasing by about 12 per cent per year totalling about

Box 3.2   A case study of Monsanto

John Francis Queeny established the Monsanto company in 1901 to produce products for the food and pharmaceutical industries. Naming the company after the maiden name of his wife, Queeny's first commercial product was the sugar substitute saccharin which was supplied in its entirety to the growing soft drink company Coca-Cola. Over the next decades, the product range expanded to include caffeine and vanillin (1904), aspirin (1917) and phenol (1919). From the 1930s, the company expanded further through the acquisition of a number of chemicals companies in the US and abroad, the supply of a diverse range of industries (e.g. rubber, textiles, paper, leather, soaps), as well as natural resources. The company also purchased interests in plastics and resins that, together with existing operations, gave Monsanto an important industrial role during the Second World War (for example in the Manhattan Project). From 1945 to 1969 the company continued to expand its operations by opening offices worldwide, creating subsidiary companies, acquiring other companies, and diversifying its product lines to include acrylic fiber, nylon, maleic anhydride (for reinforced fibreglass), petrochemicals, silicon, Astro Turf®, herbicides and seeds.

By the 1970s, Monsanto Company had become a complex collection of companies with operations in a large number of countries and sales of over US$1 billion. In 1972, under John W. Hanley as president, a re-evaluation of corporate strategy was undertaken that led to an emphasis on high-value chemicals and new directions including biotechnology. One of the first major products introduced during this period, eventually its flagship product, is the herbicide Roundup. Roundup soon became the world's number one herbicide with sales of US$2.6 billion in 2000 (48% of total company sales).

The 1980s were marked by the beginnings of biotechnology applications, most notably advances in the genetic modification of plants. This led to the further acquisition of seed, pharmaceutical and life sciences companies, but also the restructuring of the company and sale of several non-strategic businesses. Notably, G. D. Searle & Co. was acquired in 1985 and the NutraSweet Company was separated from it in 1986. Biotechnology assumed a more central role from the 1990s with the sale of Posilac (bovine somatotropic) in 1993, 'Roundup Ready' soybeans, potatoes and cotton from 1995, Roundup Ready corn from 1998, and further acquisition and collaborative agreements in the life sciences areas (Monsanto 2000b). Since the mid 1990s, Monsanto has extended its global dominance of the agricultural sector with the continued purchase of local seed companies throughout the world in order to dominate many domestic markets. For example, the company is now the largest foreign-owned agro-industry company in India. Importantly, it is the market leader in the sale of genetically modified seeds, with Monsanto GM seeds accounting for an estimated 94% of the total area planted in commercial transgenic crops (Gillam 2001).

Today, Monsanto Corporation is the most profitable agro-industrial corporation in the world with net sales of US$5.5 billion in 2000. In March 2000 Monsanto merged with Pharmacia & Upjohn to form Pharmacia

Box 3.2 continued

Corporation as a result of financial pressures from lawsuits, unexpected controversy over the safety of GM foods, and falling share prices. In October
2000 Monsanto was restructured to focus on agricultural products (notably
Roundup and biotechnology products) separately from Pharmacia
Corporation. The company remains strongly committed to GM applications,
stating that '[g]lobal acceptance of biotechnology would give us the potential for unprecedented growth' (Monsanto 2000a). It remains on the cutting
edge of 'life sciences' that could be used to mould new generations of crops,
drugs, chemicals and industrial materials.

Source: Gillam C. (2001b), 'Gene Giants Criticized at World Ag Forum', Organic
Consumers Association, <www.purefood.org/monsanto/toomuchpower.cfm>
(accessed 27 July 2001); Monsanto Company (2000a), *2000 Annual Report* (St
Louis: Monsanto Company); and Monsanto Company (2000b), 'Company
Timeline/History', St Louis, 2000b, <www.monsanto.com/monsanto/about_us/
company_timeline/default.htm> (accessed 27 July 2001).

12,000 out of about two million farms nationwide by 1997, most of
them small-scale producers. According to a recent USDA study,
certified organic cropland more than doubled from 1992 to 1997. Two
organic livestock sectors, eggs and dairy products, grew even faster. The
intensity of farming methods, aside from the ethical concerns, can
increase the risk of ill-health in the plants and animals raised which, in
turn, may pose a health risk to human populations. A notable example
is the crisis surrounding bovine spongiform encephalopathy (BSE) and
its human form, variant Creutzfeldt-Jakob disease (vCJD). Intensive
farming methods, which included the feeding of ruminant-based feeds
to cattle, was found to be the root cause of the outbreak in the UK. The
use of genetically modified organisms (GMOs) in agriculture has
elicited widespread concerns. While risks to health have not been
supported by the scientific evidence so far, the environmental consequences are more controversial. One exception has been the use of the
herbicide Roundup to fight the illicit drug trade in Colombia, which
has led to protests over potential health effects on indigenous peoples
(Bigwood 2001). More indirectly, the intensification of food production is leading to the displacement of small-scale local producers
which, in turn, has socioeconomic consequences.

Alongside food production, consumption patterns can be described
as increasingly global in nature. The historical changes to human diet
and nutrition, the so-called 'nutrition transition', can be described in

terms of five broad patterns (Table 3.2). In general, most societies have moved from small communities to larger rural and then urban-based communities. Only a few isolated communities today remain at Pattern 1 (such as the Yamamama Indians in the Brazilian Amazon rainforest). A substantial population in subSaharan Africa, Asia and Latin America remain reliant on the subsistence farming of Pattern 2, including the ever-present threat of food insecurity. Others find themselves in Pattern 3 where there is greater food security and an improving diet. Pattern 4 describes populations in industrialized countries and the relatively affluent elsewhere who have access to an abundance of food. Recent studies of growing rates of obesity among adults and children (see Chapter 5 for a discussion of the cognitive dimensions of these dietary changes) reflect the increase in so-called diseases of affluence arising in large part from over-nutrition. Finally, there is a small but growing number of health-conscious individuals comprising Pattern 5 who seek, and can afford, to adopt healthy eating patterns including the consumption of low-fat, high-fibre and organic foods.

The globalization of food consumption refers to the adoption of the 'Western high-income model' of food consumption characterized by Pattern 4 (Popkin 1994). Lang (1997: 176) laments the 'export of Northern [American] diets to the South' as a form of 'dietary burgeriza-tion' of local food consumption patterns. Importantly, this transition is not following national boundaries alone or indeed at all. While disaggregated data are limited, it appears that more complex patterns of change are occurring that cut across countries, most notably linked to socioeconomic status and urbanization. In Asia, this transition is especially notable in countries undergoing rapid industrialization. Traditionally, Asian diets are high in grains, fruits and vegetables, and low in meat and dairy products. In countries as diverse as South Korea, China, Japan, India and Thailand, the growing middle classes have increased their consumption of animal products and high fat foods, while adopting lifestyles low in physical activity. A further breakdown of this trend shows that urban dwellers, the relatively mobile, younger age group and higher socioeconomic status are all linked to dietary shifts. In other parts of the world, evidence of similar transitions is coming to light. In New Delhi, India between 30 and 40 per cent of adults of high socioeconomic status are obese, figures beginning to be comparable to the UK and US. In South Africa, shifts in diet are associ-ated with the proportion of time an individual spends living in an urban environment (Popkin 1994: 292–3).

Table 3.2   Patterns in the nutrition transition

Pattern	Features
1. Collecting food	*Hunter-gatherer period* High carbohydrates, fibre and animal protein (from wild animal meat) Low in total fat (particularly saturated fat) Tall stature and lean Few nutritional deficiencies Low life expectancy with low fertility and high mortality High rates of infectious disease with no epidemics
2. Famine	*Subsistence agricultural system* Diet less varied and subject to episodic famine (food insecurity) High carbohydrates and fibre, low animal protein Low in total fat Reduced stature by about four inches, and lean Emergence of nutritional deficiency diseases (women and children) Low life expectancy with high fertility, infant and maternal mortality High rates of infectious disease with epidemics
3. Receding famine	*More highly developed agricultural system/early industrialization* Diet still less varied but greater food security High carbohydrates, fibre, fruits and vegetables, animal proteins Low in total fat Increasing stature and lean Some nutritional deficiencies disappear Increasing life expectancy (40s–50s) with static fertility High rates of infectious disease with epidemics
4. Degenerative disease	*Industrialization and urbanization* Diet more varied High in total fat, cholesterol, sugar and refined carbohydrates Low in polyunsaturated fatty acids and fibre Taller stature and increased percentage body fat Problems of overnutrition appear such as obesity, diabetes, CHD Increasing life expectancy (60s–70s) with low fertility Low rates of infectious disease, increased incidence of chronic diseases

contd

Table 3.2 Patterns in the nutrition transition – *continued*

Pattern	Features
5. Behavioural change	*Post-industrialization, urban professionals* Diet highly varied High in fruits and vegetables, complex carbohydrates, polyunsaturated fatty acids, fibre, 'functional' foods Low in fat and refined foods Taller stature and reduced percentage body fat Increasing life expectancy (70s–80s) with low fertility Low rates of infectious disease and chronic diseases

Source: Adapted from B. Popkin, 'The Nutrition Transition in Low-Income Countries: An Emerging Crisis', *Nutrition Review*, 1994, 52(9): 285–98.

The relationship between socioeconomic status and diet, however, is not as straightforward as it initially appears and the relative cost of certain foods is also an important factor. Low-income groups in high-income countries tend to have Pattern 4 diets, and low-income households are more likely to be obese than higher-income ones. An inverse relationship between obesity and income is predicted to occur in a growing number of countries during the first decade of the twenty-first century, particularly in countries with large conglomerates of urban poor. In Brazil, the prevalence of obesity among women is now comparable to the US. Rates of childhood obesity in emerging economies are also rising so rapidly that they will soon reach the epidemic levels already found in the US. An important factor behind these trends is the relative cost of fats. In 1962 a diet deriving 20 per cent of energy from fat was associated with a GNP of US$1900. In 1993 the same diet was associated with a GNP of US$900 (both in 1993 dollars). This decline in cost is explained by revolutionary changes in the production and processing of oilseed-based fats (notably soyabean oil), the development of high-yield oilseeds, and improved methods of processing and refining (Drewnowski and Popkin 1997). As a result, the shift to high-fat diets and 'Western' eating habits, once restricted to high-income countries and the relatively well off, is now occurring in countries with lower levels of GNP and among lower-income groups. Drewnowski and Popkin (1997:41) predict a global convergence of diets towards a higher proportion of energy derived from fats (30 per cent).

Overall, trends in food production and consumption patterns, and the associated health impacts they bring, reflect changes to the spatial dimension of globalization. Traditional development theory holds that economic growth leads to diversification of food sources, improved quantity and quality of food, and increased food security, all of which contribute to better health. More recent research on global trends in diet and nutrition suggest worrying trends that follow patterns of global change. More detailed analysis of these emerging transnational patterns suggest that analysis of the nutrition transition cannot be limited to nationally based aggregates, but must seek to capture new spatial patterns, as well as patterns that are nonterritorially based.

3.3.3 The globalization of the tobacco industry

[T]he international market opportunity is what will keep us a growth company for many years to come.
Geoffrey Bible, CEO of Phillip Morris (as quoted in Somasundaram 1996)

Record revenues, record volumes, and record profits...
Martin Broughton, Chairman of BAT (2001)

Unlike the pharmaceutical and food industries, the tobacco industry markets a product that is known to be harmful to human health. The scientific evidence on the harmful effects of tobacco use has been recognized by the medical community since the 1950s, and is finally acknowledged by the industry itself after decades of denial. Today, 1.1 billion people smoke, about one-third of the world's population over the age of fifteen. Smoking-related diseases, led by lung cancer, bronchitis, emphysema and heart disease, are responsible for one in ten deaths worldwide or 4.9 million people annually. Smoking is now the greatest preventable cause of death and disability.[3] Mortality from tobacco is expected to rise to 8–10 million deaths annually by 2030, 70 per cent of these deaths to occur in the developing world (WHO 1997b).

While tobacco has been traded internationally for hundreds of years, as described in Chapter 2, the geographical distribution and reach, and the scale of this trade, has changed markedly in recent decades. In a number of ways, these changes are closely linked to processes of globalization. First, the decline of traditional markets in high-income countries has led transnational tobacco companies (TTCs) to search for new markets worldwide. As such, there has been a clear shift in industry attention from high- to low- and middle-income countries, as well as population groups that have so far been 'underserved', notably women, young people and even children. Already, these efforts are paying off. The tobacco industry has long been a highly profitable industry, but it has seen unprecedented growth since the late 1980s. Between 1989 and 1999 Phillip Morris's international revenues increased 226 per cent (to US$27.4 billion) and profits by 400 per cent (to US$5.05 billion). Overseas sales of Japan Tobacco have risen for seven consecutive quarters from mid 1999 while domestic sales declined (Link and Rossel 2001:18). Similarly, BAT reported record profits year-on-year since the late 1990s, with a 36 per cent rise in profits between 2000 and 2001. This included particular gains in the Asia-Pacific (15 per cent) and America-Pacific (16 per cent) regions over the single year (BAT 2001a). Smoking among women and girls is increasing rapidly, with current figures of 200 million female smokers expected to triple in the next 25 years (WHO 1999a). Overall, the developing world is expected to provide 85 per cent of the world's smokers by 2025, an increase from the current 72 per cent (Hammond 1998).

The pursuit of new markets has led to major restructuring within the tobacco industry towards consolidation around a small number of large companies (Table 3.3). With the exception of the China National Tobacco Corporation (CNTC), all are transnational entities with operational reach in all the major regions of the world. Seeking access to new markets, 'Big Tobacco' has systematically bought up local companies or built strategic alliances with domestic producers. Along with cigarette manufacturers, TTCs have developed strong links with local retailers, wholesalers, advertisers, mass media and tobacco farmers. This horizontal and vertical integration of the industry has been part

Table 3.3 The world's three largest tobacco companies (2000)

	Phillip Morris International (PMI)	British American Tobacco (BAT)	Japan Tobacco
Cigarette production (% of world total)	16.5	15.0	8.1
Cigarettes produced in 2000 (billions)	887.3	807.0	447.9
Number of brands		300	190
Number of countries with operations	180	180	170
Number of countries with factories		64	

Source: E. Link and S. Rossel (2001), 'Global tobacco: where cigarette manufacturers roam', *Tobacco Journal International*, 6 (November/December): 17–20.

of what Yach and Bettcher (2000) describe as 'the homogenization of the global tobacco industry' by industry strategists, allowing worldwide sourcing of inputs, access to cheap labour, and greater economies of scale in production (the global marketing strategies of the tobacco industry are discussed in Chapter 5). As a result, TTCs have become among the largest economic entities in the world. In 1998, the three largest TTCs together had revenues of more than US$88 billion, more than the GDP of countries such as Ireland and New Zealand. The largest, Phillip Morris, is ranked 28th among the world's top 200 corporations with revenues of US$61.7 billion and profits of US$7.675 billion (Anderson and Cavanagh 2000).

Where national governments have been resistant to the increased presence of foreign companies, either from concern for protecting domestic producers or public health, TTCs have been highly effective at using the platform of trade liberalization to exert pressure. Beginning in the mid 1980s, this has been achieved bilaterally through the US Trade Representative who pressed Japan, South Korea, Thailand and Taiwan to open up their markets to American imports or face retaliatory trade sanctions. All of these countries had imposed higher tariffs on imported than domestic cigarettes, or banned imports alto-gether. With the exception of Thailand, they eventually complied which resulted in a 10 per cent increase overall in smoking rates (Chaloupka and Laixuthai 1996). For the most promising market of all, the Chinese market, the 'carrot' of WTO membership helped secure a bilateral agreement between the US and China in November 1999 requiring China to reduce tariffs on cigarettes from 65 per cent to 25 per cent by January 2004. The US government was not alone in pro-moting trade in tobacco products during this period. BAT maintained a close relationship with successive Conservative administrations of the British government throughout the 1980s and 1990s, with leading ministers playing a prominent role in trade missions to secure new markets for the industry (Kessler 2001).

As well as bilateral negotiations, TTCs have been successful at pene-trating world markets using multilateral trade agreements. The Uruguay Round of the General Agreement on Trade and Tariffs (GATT) included, for the first time, agreements to liberalize trade in unmanu-factured tobacco. The 1992 ruling by GATT against the government of Thailand, on the grounds of equal treatment of domestic and foreign cigarette manufacturers, further demonstrated the primacy given to trade over public health objectives (Chantornvong and McCargo 2001). Under WTO agreements to reduce tariff and nontarriff barriers,

---

Box 3.3   A case study of British American Tobacco

British American Tobacco (BAT) was formed in 1902 as a joint venture between the Imperial Tobacco Company in the UK and the American Tobacco Company (ATC) of the US. The agreement arose from an intense trade war within the industry that led the two companies to agree not to trade in the other's domestic market, and to assign trademarks, export businesses and overseas subsidiaries to the joint venture. With James 'Buck' Duke as chairman, the new company established operations in a wide range of countries including Canada, China, Germany, South Africa and Australia. By 1910 its operations extended to the West Indies, India, Sri Lanka, East Africa, Malaysia and Nigeria. It was through these early roots that BAT has become a more global concern today than any other major tobacco company.

In 1911 ATC was broken up and its shares in BAT were divested and acquired by British investors. In this way BAT became a British company that was now free to conduct its business independently anywhere in the world except in the UK where Imperial Tobacco remained protected by territorial agreements. Over the next decades, BAT acquired companies in still more countries: Souza Cruz in Brazil (1914), the overseas business of Ardath Tobacco (1925), Brown & Williamson in the US (1927), Haus Bergmann Zigarettenfabrik in Germany (1932) and the overseas business of Benson & Hedges (1956). During this period, growth in sales remained strong, buoyed by its international brands State Express and Benson & Hedges.

In 1961 shareholders approved the company's diversification, and over the next three decades BAT expanded into paper and pulp, cosmetics, retailing (e.g. Argos, Saks Fifth Avenue) and financial services (e.g. Allied Dunbar, Eagle Star, Farmers). By 1970 BAT companies were manufacturing in 140 factories in 50 countries. A reorganization in the 1970s led to the creation of the new holding company, BAT Industries, to coordinate its diverse business concerns. The covenant with Imperial Tobacco was revoked in 1972 and its remaining shareholdings were sold, leaving BAT with exclusive ownership of its original brands. Between 1971 and 1981 tobacco profits tripled to more than £463 million. Then the end of the Cold War provided an opportunity to expand international operations, particularly into eastern and central Europe, and the Far East, beginning with the purchase of Hungary's largest cigarette manufacturer Pécsi in 1992. In 1999 BAT merged with Rothmans International, then the fourth largest tobacco company in the world, and in 2000 the company acquired full ownership of Canada's largest cigarette company, Imperial Tobacco.

Today, the BAT Group of companies is the second largest tobacco group in the world with a market share of 15% and annual shipments of more than 800 billion cigarettes. Operating profits grew 27% in 2000 (£2575 million), and paid about US$20 billion in excise tax and duties worldwide. The group has 87,000 employees, 86 factories in 64 countries, and an active business presence in 180 markets. Notably, its operations are organized into five regions (America-Pacific, Asia-Pacific, Latin America, Europe and Amesca), based around global, regional and local brand names. Its declared

---

Box 3.3 continued

aim is to achieve global leadership through increasing its share of the premium and 'lights' segments.

Source: H. Cox (2000), *The Global Cigarette, Origins and Evolution of British American Tobacco* (Oxford: Oxford University Press); BAT (2001c), 'Our history', <www.bat.co.uk> (accessed 31.07.01); and BAT (2001a), *Annual Review and Summary of Financial Statements 2000* (London: BAT Industries, 2001).

---

the global trade in tobacco products will be further facilitated. Regional trade agreements, such as the EU, NAFTA, Association of South-East Asian Nations (ASEAN), Common Market of East and Southern Africa (COMESA), Economic Community of West African States (ECOWAS), Common Market of the South (MERCOSUR) and Organization of American States (OAS) all have provisions for liberalizing trade in goods and services, including tobacco (Bettcher et al. 2001). Economic analysis of the public health impact of such policies has shown a rise in cigarette consumption as a result of freer trade, with the biggest impact on low- and middle-income countries (Jha and Chaloupka 2000).

Finally, it is important to note the significant transborder problem of cigarette smuggling in the context of the changing geography of the tobacco industry. Smuggling occurs when cigarettes manufactured legally are exported without domestic taxes for sale abroad. These untaxed cigarettes are then illegally brought back into the producer country to be sold at a cheaper price on the black market. It is estimated that 6 per cent of the total number of cigarettes consumed worldwide are smuggled (Jha and Chaloupka 2000). The scale of smuggling operations, complex transborder networks of supply and distribution that exists, the central role of organized crime in such activities, the laundering of financial proceeds through the global financial system, and difficulties of national authorities in preventing such activities, make tobacco smuggling an issue that defies national boundaries. Furthermore, there is growing evidence that TTCs are themselves implicated in smuggling operations, resulting in litigation and public investigations in the US, UK and elsewhere (Abrams 2000; Joosens 2002).

The spatial dimensions of the tobacco industry, in short, are increasingly defined by global parameters. The changing structure of the industry, operating strategies, and public health impact of its activities in recent decades are intimately linked to processes of globalization as a whole.

3.4 Global environmental change and health

> *From the point of view of other organisms, humankind ... resembles an acute epidemic disease, whose occasional lapses into less virulent forms of behaviour have never yet sufficed to permit any really stable, chronic relationship to establish itself.*
>
> McNeill, *Plagues and People* (1976: 22).

> *It's a tragedy, but it's just part and parcel of what we're doing not only to the animals but to ourselves.*
>
> Jane Goodall on the hunting of great apes in Central Africa, as quoted in Astill (2001)

The links between global environmental change and health demonstrate well the spatial dimensions of globalization. As defined in Chapter 1, global environmental change can be natural or human-induced (anthropogenic). Natural environmental changes have occurred long before the human species evolved and will continue to do so regardless of our actions. For example, periods of glaciation and inter-glaciation over the history of the planet when average temperatures regionally and globally, sea levels and patterns of flora and fauna change over time. What is distinct about recent decades is the unprecedented degree of anthropogenic environmental change that is occurring, developments arising as part of processes of globalization. It is these latter phenomena that raise new and alarming implications for spatial patterns of health and disease.

In the most basic sense, human health is dependent on the Earth's natural biophysical systems. Degradation of these systems – climate, stratospheric ozone, biodiversity, terrestrial and marine food-producing ecosystems, and great cycles of water, nitrogen and sulphur – to a point that human life cannot be sustained would be the ultimate threat to health. For this reason, the First Assessment Report of the Intergovernmental Panel on Climate Change (IPCC) stated in 1990 that '[t]he sustained health of human populations requires the continued integrity of Earth's natural systems' (as quoted in McMichael et al. 1999). This begins with a holistic approach that recognizes the interconnectedness of all of these biophysical systems, and what McMichael et al. (1999) call an ecological approach that links globalization with environmental sustainability and human health. Such an approach redefines territorial (state) boundaries, either in terms of subsystems that form part of the larger whole, or views them as irrelevant where global-level systems are at play. In either case, global environmental change challenges us to rethink orthodox concepts of territorial space.

On the whole, there is worrying evidence that the human species is causing unprecedented, and in some cases irreversible, damage to the natural environment through the burning of fossil fuels, unsustainable use of natural resources, destruction of habitats, degradation of air and water quality, and deforestation. The scale and pace of these environmental changes has increased over the past three decades, closely linked to processes of globalization. The Living Planet Index, an annual measure developed by the Worldwide Fund for Nature (WWF) of the changing state of the world's natural ecosystems (forests, freshwater ecosystems, oceans and coast), for example, shows that humans have destroyed 31 per cent of the natural world since 1970 (WWF 2002). The driving force has been the emerging global economy that has encouraged the globalization of unsustainable production and consumption practices. The volume of FDI has grown almost fifteenfold since 1970, reaching US$644 billion in 1998, while the number of TNCs has grown over the same period from 7000 to 60,000 in 2000 (French 2000). There has been an upsurge in trade and investment in resources such as forestry, mining and fossil fuels. Human consumption has doubled over the last 25 years and continues to accelerate (WWF 2000).

Scientific understanding of the health consequences of different types of global environmental change is growing (Table 3.4). Degradation of the natural environment locally, for example, can have health consequences by affecting food production, clean air and water supplies, or exposure to hazardous substances. On a global level, changes to the natural environment can have similar but more widespread consequences for human health. Global climate change, for instance, is contributing to the warming of air and water temperatures that, in turn, impact on the habitability of certain locations because of flooding or drought. More catastrophically, many scientists fear serious and potentially irreversible disruptions of the complex and interrelated ecology that sustains all life on earth.

These concerns are supported by worrying trends in health and disease. One major area of concern is the impact of global climate change on the epidemiology of certain diseases such as malaria, yellow fever and dengue

Table 3.4   Summary of the potential health impacts of global environmental change

Global environmental change	Specific effects	Potential health impact
Global climate change	Warming of average world and regional temperatures from greenhouse gases	Increase in incidence of vector-borne diseases including malaria, lymphatic filariasis, onchocerciasis, schistosomiasis, African trypanosomiasis, Leishmaniasis, dracunculiasis, arboviral diseases (dengue, yellow fever, Japanese encephalitis)
	Increase in extreme weather events such as floods, hurricanes, excessive rainfall	Increase in incidence of natural disasters, disruption of food production, increase in risk of waterborne diseases such as cholera, contamination of water supplies, creation of breeding sites for disease vectors, forced migration of people and increased risk to infectious disease
Deforestation and forest degradation	Destruction of habitats and related human activities; nutrient depletion; use of land for cash crops; contribution to global climate change and loss of biodiversity	Impacts on ecology of vectors and epidemiology of vector-borne diseases; production of products that have adverse health impacts (e.g. tobacco)
Loss of biodiversity	Extinction of plant and animal species	Loss of plants and compounds for potential use in medicines; loss of animal species linked to human disease; change in ecology of vector-borne diseases from composition of species, predator-prey relationship and habitats
Change in water quality	Poisoning of water supplies with toxic substances	Increase in risk of water-borne diseases; lack of clean drinking water

Table 3.4   Summary of the potential health impacts of global environmental change – *continued*

Global environmental change	Specific effects	Potential health impact
	(e.g. arsenic, lead); major water projects lowering water tables; depletion of freshwater aquifers	
Change in air quality	Greater presence of particles of damaging substances in air such as lead, asbestos, tobacco smoke	Effects on haeme synthesis and other biochemical processes, impairment of psychological and neurobehavioural functions; damage to central nervous system; respiratory disorders; lung cancer
Production and exposure to harmful substances	Production and use of pesticides, chemicals, poisons, PCBs	

Source: J. Patz, P. Epstein, T. Burke and J. Balbus (1996), 'Global Climate Change and Emerging Infectious Diseases', *Journal of the American Medical Association*, 275(3): 217–23; S. Tong, Y. von Schirnding and T. Prapamontol (2000), 'Environmental lead exposure: a public health problem of global dimensions', *Bulletin of the World Health Organization*, 78(9): 1068–77; and A. J. McMichael and A. Haines (1997), 'Global climate change: the potential effects on health', *British Medical Journal*, 315: 805–9.

fever. Climate change may have direct effects on vector and parasite biology and distribution, and indirect effects on regional food supply and human migration patterns that can alter susceptibility to infectious agents (Patz et al. 1996). A good example is malaria. As described in Chapter 2, malaria has plagued humankind for thousands of years. Historically, the disease has been spread by naturally occurring changes in temperature, as well as patterns of population mobility and settlement (such as certain agricultural practices). For example, malaria was introduced to Guam during the Vietnam War by American aircraft using the island as a refuelling station. The resurgence of malaria from the late twentieth century has spurred renewed international efforts to control the disease in populations currently at risk. Recent research suggests that human-induced climate change in future will affect the length of the transmission season in many areas and, to a limited extent, the size of areas suitable for malaria transmission. It is estimated that the number of additional people at risk due to climate change by 2080 will be up to 320 million for *Plasmodium falciparum* and 200 million for *P. vivax* depending on the climate scenario used (Martens et al. 1999).

The health impacts of global environmental change are not always readily apparent, making it difficult to empirically demonstrate causal relationships. A good example is the logging industry in Central Africa that is opening up new areas of virgin rainforests. A lucrative offshoot of this industry is the capture and sale of so-called 'bush meat': indigenous animals, many of them rare, for human consumption. The great apes, many of them protected species, are among the most sought-after animals in this new trade, and it is expected that they will become extinct within 10–15 years (Astill 2001). Among species indigenous to the region are a rare species of chimpanzee that scientists believe may help explain the origins of HIV/AIDS. The expected extinction of this species of chimpanzee may threaten our ability to understand the origins of the disease and hence develop effective vaccines and treatments (Gao et al. 1999).

Another example of an indirect consequence is the outbreak of foot (hoof) and mouth disease among sheep and cattle in the UK in February 2001. Some scientists believe the cause of the outbreak was a cloud of infected dust from the Sahara desert. The frequency of storms carrying dust from Africa to Europe is increasing as a result of climate change. A decline in rainfall is leading to increased desertification and hence the production of more dust clouds. As one scientist stated, 'There is no sewage treatment or proper garbage disposal there – so the soil is heavily infected with microbes and faeces' (Dr Eugene Shinn as quoted in McKie 2001). Analysis of dust clouds has found a wide range of plant and animal pathogens. The clouds are funnelled westward to the Caribbean by the summer trade winds and northward to Europe during winter. Scientists are concerned that the clouds may be responsible for other epidemics including asthma outbreaks in Barbados and Puerto Rico, and a disease destroying Caribbean coral reefs (Shinn et al. 2000).

The health impacts of global environmental change illustrate well the need to rethink our perception and experience of territorial space. Perhaps more than any other type of global change, environmental changes demonstrate the interconnected nature of the world as a whole. It is the 'common fate' that we share in protecting the Earth's capacity to sustain life that creates the imperative to critically reflect on what effects globalization is having on the natural world.

3.5   Global demographic change and health

There is almost no place on Earth that cannot be reached by a migrant or
a product, within 1–2 days of travel.

MacPherson (2001)

A change closely related to the above concerns demographic trends
arising as a consequence of globalization. Global demographic change
includes the size of human populations, and patterns of mobility and
settlement. Human populations have grown steadily throughout
history, but growth has occurred at an unprecedented rate over the
past two centuries (Table 3.5). Between 8000 BC and 1750, populations
doubled every one thousand years. From 1750 to 1950, agricultural
development and the Industrial Revolution contributed to a doubling
time of less than forty years. Today, world population increases at a
rate of 250,000 per day or around eight million people per month.
Depending on average fertility (number of children per woman), it is
estimated that world population will stabilize at around 10–12.5 billion
by 2050 (Bioembergen 1997; Cohen 1996).

As well as population growth, patterns of human mobility are changing fundamentally. The advent of mass transportation by air, sea, rail
and road has enabled people to travel further and more frequently
than ever before. The average number of kilometres travelled daily by
French nationals between 1800 and 2000, for example, increased more
than a thousandfold (Grubler and Nakicenovic 1991, as cited in Wilson
1995). In the US, revenue passenger-miles for air travel increased 90 per
cent between 1980 and 1995 (ICAF 1996). The reasons why people
travel help distinguish forms of population mobility. Tourism is a term
used in official statistics to denote travel of less than twelve months by
people permanently resident in a country other than their destination
including for study, business and holidaymaking. Migration, in contrast, refers to travel for at least one year to a destination country
including emigrants, asylum seekers, displaced people or refugees. It is
notable that different national and international authorities use
varying categories and definitions, making comparative analysis
difficult.

Despite limitations in available data, it is clear that the general
picture is one of increased population mobility of various forms since
the late twentieth century. According to the World Tourism
Organization (WTO), total international arrivals worldwide reached
699 million in 2000, an annual increase of 7.9 per cent. The average

Table 3.5 The historical growth of world population

Date	*Estimated world population*
1.6 million years ago	100,000
200,000 years ago	10,000*
35,000 BC	1–5 million
10,000 BC	10 million
7000 BC	10–21 million
2000 BC	46–47 million
At the time of Christ	93–230 million
AD 1000	185–345 million
AD 1500	366–540 million
AD 1600	500 million
AD 1750	750 million
AD 1800	887–907 million
AD 1850	1158–1170 million
AD 1900	1656–1710 million
AD 1950	2515–2812 million
AD 1990	5328 million
AD 2000	6261–6265 million
AD 2050	10,019–12,500 million
AD 2100	11,186–12,034 million
AD 2150	11,543–12,648 million
AD 2200	11,600–12,946 million
AD 2500	13,536–14,000 million

* Genetic research on the origins of humankind suggests that all humans descended from a group of about 10,000 *Homo sapiens* who lived in Africa about 200,000 years ago. Earlier population estimates include other *Homo* species.

Source: Compiled from S. Kapitsa (1997), 'A model of world population growth as an experiment in systematic research', *Voprosy Statistiki*, 8: 46–57; Bioembergen N. (1997), 'A discussion of human population growth', *Carrying Capacity Network Focus*, 7(1): 10–14; Cohen J. (1996), 'Maximum occupancy', *American Demographics*, 18(2): 50–1; and R. Gallant (1990), *The Peopling of Planet Earth: Human Population Growth through the Ages* (New York: Macmillan).

increase in tourist arrivals over the ten years to 2000 was 4.3 per cent per annum. As well as more frequent travel, tourists are travelling further afield. The number of long-haul travellers is expected to reach 377 million by 2020 (World Tourism Organization 2001). There has also been a substantial increase in the number of people working legally or illegally in other countries. In 1965 an estimated 75 million people worked as migrants. By the late 1990s this had increased to 130 million (ILO 2000). Similarly, a dramatic increase in refugees has occurred over the past 40 years. In 1961 there was an estimated 1.4 million refugees. By the early 1990s this had increased to about

20 million with another 30 million internally displaced persons world-wide (IOM as cited in Wilson 1995). Refugee numbers peaked in 1995 at 27.4 million, declining to 21.8 million by 2000 (UNHCR 2001). Finally, it is estimated that around 4 million people are the victims of human trafficking each year (USAID 1999), earning profits for traffickers of US$7 billion annually (IOM 1998). There are, of course, certain key pressure points. More than 800,000 people cross the 2100-mile US–Mexican border legally each day, with at least an additional 5000 illegally. Mexicans comprise nearly half of the 8 million illegal immigrants in the US. Consequently, the American government spends US$2 billion annually to patrol the border (Vulliamy 2001b).

One key destination of recent human migration is cities. The greater concentration of populations in larger and larger urban areas is expected to be a continuing trend in the twenty-first century, posing new challenges for public health. By 2025 it is estimated that 61 per cent of the world's population will be living in urban areas (UNFPA 1995). By 2000 there were 22 megacities (see Table 3.6), defined as having populations exceeding 10 million inhabitants, 18 of them in low- and middle-income countries. This figure is expected to grow to 27 cities by 2015. While the populations of cities such as Tokyo, Osaka, New York, Los Angeles and Paris are expected to remain relatively stable, rapid growth rates are predicted for many cities in the developing world between 2000 and 2020, notably Jakarta (57%), Karachi (64%), Dhaka (72%), Bombay (74%) and Lagos (84%). The drivers behind urbanization are complex but the globalization of industrialization processes is a key factor. The displacement of rural workers from agricultural lands, the search for employment by the poor, and the concentration of means of production in cities all mirror developments in high-income countries from the seventeenth century. For example, maquiladores are factories in Mexico opened under special tax incentives following the NAFTA, paying triple the Mexican minimum wage. Their presence has led to the mass migration of people seeking work, resulting in a burgeoning of communities along the US–Mexican border. Similarly, special economic zones in China have transformed many small towns and villages within a short time into large thriving cities.

The establishment of towns and cities during medieval times and later the Industrial Revolution was synonymous with the rise in so-called 'crowd diseases'. Rapid population growth and increased density of communities was accompanied by a lack of sanitation and clean drinking water, and hence substantial fluctuations in population size (Harris 2001). Rapid urbanization since the late twentieth century has created similar

Table 3.6 World megacities 1975, 2000 and projections to 2015 (population in millions)

City	1975	2000	Projections to 2015
Tokyo	19.8	26.4	26.4–28.9
New York	15.9	16.6	17.4
Shanghai	11.4	14.6	17.0–18.0
Mexico City	11.2	18.1	19.2
Sao Paolo	10.0	17.8	20.4
Bombay		18.1	26.2
Lagos		13.4	23.2–24.6
Los Angeles		13.1	14.1
Kolkata		12.9	17.3
Buenos Aires		12.6	13.9–14.1
Dhaka		12.3	21.1
Calcutta		11.9 (1995)	17.3
Karachi		11.8	19.2–19.4
Delhi		11.7	16.8
Seoul		11.6 (1995)	13.0
Jakarta		11.0	17.3
Osaka		11.0	10.6–11.0
Metro Manila		10.9	14.8
Beijing		10.8	12.3–15.6
Rio de Janiero		10.6	11.9
Cairo		10.6	13.8–14.4
Paris		9.5	9.7
Istanbul			12.5
Tianjin			10.7
Hyderabad			10.5
Bangkok			10.1

Source: UNFPA (2002), *The State of the World's Population 2001* (New York: UN Population Fund), Table 1; and <www.wri.org/wri/trends/citygrow>

conditions in many parts of the developing world where shanty towns and squatter settlements have sprung up to accommodate the urban poor and transient populations. The health risks arising from such environmental conditions are well known beginning with the increased risk of infectious diseases because of a lack of access to safe drinking water and sanitation. More than one billion people worldwide do not have access to safe drinking water and more than two million deaths result from water-related diseases annually. Other hazards include physical dangers from unsafe roads and violence, indoor and outdoor air pollution, and exposure to toxic wastes (McMichael 2000).

3.6 Conclusions

This chapter has only begun to touch on the diverse ways that the spatial dimensions of globalization are relevant to human health. However, we can see from the above that orthodox delineations of territorial space do not fully capture the range of changes taking place. It is argued here that a new global geography of health is needed that goes beyond territorial boundaries defined by states, to include the reterritorialization, and even deterritorialization, of health determinants, needs and outcomes.

First, an additional global dimension to each of the determinants of health is needed. The determinants of health are now widely recognized as encompassing a broad range of factors related to: (a) individual characteristics and behaviours; (b) the physical environment; and (c) the social and economic environment. Epidemiologists have long recognized that patterns of health and disease do not necessarily follow, and determinants of health are not necessarily confined by, national boundaries. Where determinants of health are seen to be crossborder, national governments may co-operate with other governments to address health issues that affect more than one country through the WHO and other international organizations.

The challenge of understanding global health is to recognize health determinants that are *transborder* in their origin or impact; that is, determinants where territorial space is increasingly irrelevant. Public health remains strongly wedded to territorial concepts of space. The term 'tropical medicine' has its origins in European colonization. It became a specialist field based on diseases, such as malaria, that occur primarily in the tropical regions of the world, an assumption valid at the time that certain diseases occur in certain territorial locations. In a globalizing world, the validity of the term needs to be reassessed given global climate change and its impact on the habitation of certain disease vectors to new geographies, and the increase in imported cases of such diseases to non-tropical regions. The possibility that patterns of health and disease may be unrelated, at least in part, to territorial space raises the need for new thinking about medical geography. The spatial strategies conventionally used in infectious disease control assume that outbreaks of disease are geographically localized, and the task is to prevent the spread to other individuals and population groups through spatial strategies. Influenza is a good exception to the effectiveness of such strategies as described by Cliff and Hagett (1989: 343).

> the increasing flux within the human population and the exponential increase in the volume and speed of travel makes spatial containment in disease control more difficult in the late twentieth century than at any previous time in human history.

The historical emphasis on infectious diseases has led, in particular, to fields of study that embody the strong emphasis on territorial space and, in particular, on the state. Foremost is medical geography which concerns two main areas of study: (a) disease ecology that seeks to elucidate the social and environmental causes of ill-health; and (b) geography of medical care in terms of distribution and access (akin to economics and sociology). The former is closely related to epidemiology, the study of the distribution and determinants of disease frequency in humans so that they can be prevented and controlled (Jones and Moon 1987; Beaglehole and Bonita 1997: 85). Spatial analyses lie at the heart of medical geography of which there are five main approaches: (a) a cartographic approach, concerned with the mapping of spatial data; (b) a modelling approach that seeks to quantify relationships between variables; (c) a behavioural approach that seeks to understand individual decision-making; (d) a welfare approach that attempts to answer the questions of who gets what and where, and how quality of life can be improved by reform of existing society; and (e) a structuralist perspective that stresses the need to consider phemonena in relation to the totality of society (Jones and Moon 1987: 1–2).

A useful example is the spatial control strategies to infectious disease control. In a review of the latter, Cliff and Haggett (1989) classify the wide range of strategies in the following way:

(a) To disrupt the route from susceptible to recovered cases by the establishment of immunity through some variant of immunization; and
(b) To interrupt the mixing of infectives and susceptibles with protective spatial barriers by
    (i) isolating individuals or communities, or restricting the geographical movements of infected individuals by quarantine requirements; or

(ii) creating a *cordon sanitaire* in the case of animal populations whereby wholesale evacuation of areas occurs or by the destruction of those infected (as in the foot and mouth outbreak in the UK in 2001).

The latter comprises four different spatial control strategies: local elimination, defensive isolation, offensive containment, and global eradication.

Second, understanding of health needs and outcomes are predicated on the fact that health data are overwhelmingly collected according to national populations or subgroups within this population. These data are then aggregated nationally, regionally or internationally. The Global Burden of Disease (GBD) study is a well-known example of this type of data (Murray and Lopez 1996). Other examples are the *World Health Report* (WHO), *World Development Report* (World Bank), *Human Development Report* (UNDP), *State of the World's Children* (UNICEF) and *State of the World's Population* (UNFPA). All use national data (of varying quality) as building blocks to compile an overall picture of health worldwide.

The limitations of available health data are a major challenge to understanding the global dimensions of health. It is argued here that globalization is creating new 'populations' that require identification and analyses, populations that (a) do not conform along state-defined territorial boundaries; and (b) that may not even be territorially defined. The particular health needs of some of these populations are already being recognized. The health needs of women across the world, by virtue of their biology and gender, is one example. While recognizing that there may be distinctive features of women in particular countries, their female identity is the key variable that defines this population group. Using Wallerstein's world-system theory, Dyches and Rushing (1996: 1064) support sociological perspectives that shift the focus from 'how' disease develops to 'why' disease develops by directing the observer to 'recognition that health and illness are produced from the global organization of societies and the means of production and distribution of subsistence and surplus goods and services'. They argue that the study of such macrolevel determinants of health reveals new perspectives on, for example, the 'global context within which the oppression of women takes place' and 'macrolevel socioeconomic factors impacting the global status of women, including their health status'. Other global population groups undefined by territorial geography might include:

- unskilled or nonunionized labourers in special economic zones
- communities located at sea level
- undocumented migrants
- poor in slum or shanty towns in urban peripheries
- homeless
- users of illicit drugs and particularly injecting drug users
- commercial sex workers
- middle class in urban areas
- indigenous peoples
- diaspora of various ethnic groups (for example Indian, Chinese, Jews).

What defines the needs of these population groups is not their territorial location but the health impact of processes of global change on them. Their health needs are not territorially defined but are defined by their 'place' in the emerging global order. They have particular health needs that arise because of their location within the global economy or location in relation to global environmental change. It is not because they happen to live in country X or country Y. If we think about population groups in this alternative way, then how we compile data on health status and develop health interventions to meet those needs becomes very different.

Third, the traditional model of health systems focuses on the national government responsible for the health of the population within its sovereign territory. The state is the main means by which to carry out the promotion and pursuit of public health for populations under its national jurisdiction. The structure and organization of health systems throughout the world have evolved accordingly, with each national health system responsible for the health of populations within its sovereign territory. The plenary body of the World Health Organization (WHO), the World Health Assembly (WHA), is comprised of delegations (led by the ministry of health) of each member state. Almost all health data are presented in national aggregates, subnational components or combinations thereof (e.g. regional), and 'global' is widely used in the medical literature to refer to collective national data (e.g. Global Burden of Disease). However, the spatial dimension of global change challenges us to think innovatively about their impacts on health systems. How are the health systems of the present affected by globalization? How should the health systems of the future be structured?

These changes, in turn, challenge us as scholars, policy makers and practitioners to rethink how we define populations and their health needs, to re-tool ourselves with new paradigms, methods of analyses and policy responses, and to reorganize the ways in which we work collectively to promote and protect health. As described by Hardt and Negri (2000), the flip side of the deterritorialized global space is the opportunity to find human commonalities. When we stop worrying about defining and defending territorial spaces, we are liberated to think about shared values of freedom, social justice, human rights and responsibilities, and creativity.

The above points to the need for a global geography of health, both analytically and empirically, as a core aspect of globalization. There is a need to identify population groups in a way that captures the contours of globalizing processes, and new patterns of health and disease that are emerging individually and collectively. The changing territorial nature of health questions how health can be understood in relation to this emerging global geography. While state-defined territorial geography remains important, it is increasingly insufficient in itself to ensure the protection and promotion of human health.

Key Readings

Aron J. L. and J. A Patz eds. *Ecosystem Change and Public Health, A Global Perspective* (Baltimore: Johns Hopkins University Press).

Lee K. and R. Dodgson (2000), 'Globalisation and cholera: Implications for global governance', *Global Governance*, 6(2): 213–36.

Scholte J. A. (2000), 'What is "Global" about Globalization' in *Globalization, a Critical Introduction* (London: Macmillan – now Palgrave Macmillan): 41–61.

4

The Temporal Dimension of Global Health

'If you knew Time as well as I do,' said the Hatter, 'you wouldn't talk about wasting it. It's him.'
'I don't know what you mean,' said Alice.
'Of course, you don't!' the Hatter said, tossing his head contemptuously. 'I daresay you never even spoke to Time!'
'Perhaps not,' Alice cautiously replied; 'but I know I have to beat time when I learn music.'
'Ah! That accounts for it,' said the Hatter. 'He won't stand beating.'
Lewis Carroll, *Alice's Adventures in Wonderland* (1865)

4.1 Introduction

The temporal dimension of global change concerns how we perceive and experience time. Globalization is changing the timeframe of many types of social interaction, changes that are closely linked to the spatial dimension described in the previous chapter. In many ways, the speed at which we live our lives is accelerating. We feel it in our daily work and in our personal lives – the constant pressures of limited time. Life seems increasingly like a race against the clock, with more and more people to see, more things to do. In other ways, time seems to be decelerating. Large bureaucracies have come to symbolize modern institutions, slowed by their sheer size and complexity. Our efforts to move from one place to another are prevented at times by traffic jams and the prospect of gridlock on the main roads of many large cities. Our ability to obtain information may only be a few keyboard taps away, but our ability to digest the mountains of information available remains essentially static.

This chapter explores how changes to our perceptions and experiences of time, as a consequence of global change, have implications for

104

human health. In many ways, our capacity to promote and protect public health is affected by the time available to us. How long does it take for health risks and opportunities to manifest themselves? How quickly can we mobilize the appropriate decisions, resources and actions to respond to a health need? What 'window of opportunity' do we have to effectively control an infectious disease and stop it from raging like a forest fire out of control? How long do we have to produce effective health interventions, such as vaccines and antimicrobials, to meet the health needs of today and tomorrow? What does sustainability mean in the context of short and long-term health needs? Following a discussion of the temporal dimension of global change, these types of questions are explored in relation to selected health issues. As with previous chapters, the topics explored are illustrative rather than comprehensive, serving to demonstrate the complex links between globalization and health.

4.2 Speeding up, slowing down: the pace of global change

> *How we construct and use our time, in the end, defines the texture and quality of our existence.*
>
> Robert Levine, *A Geography of Time* (1997)

As described in Chapter 3, globalization is having unprecedented impacts on how we perceive and experience physical space, in some cases redefining the way we organize and interact within territorial boundaries, in other cases, rendering them irrelevant. Closely linked to these spatial changes are the timeframes in which human interaction takes place. In many ways, social interaction is a function of physical distance, with the greater the territorial distance, the longer the timeframe for interaction to take place. However, as Scholte (2000: 48–9) writes, 'the world has long been "shrinking", as territorial distances have been covered in progressively shorter time intervals'. The advent of progressively faster, higher-volume and cheaper communication and transportation technologies have been at the heart of this 'shrinkage'. If place is no longer territorially fixed, as a strict definition of globalization asserts, then 'territorial distance is covered in effectively no time … Hence globality in the sense of transworld simultaneity and instantaneity – in the sense of a single world space – refers to something distinctive'.

In other words, this delinking of time and space means that social interaction is no longer necessarily a function of territorial distance.

The cost of sending electronic mail (e-mail), for example, is not dependent on the geographical distance between the sender and receiver, but the technology used and the nature (size, graphics versus text) of the message itself. The growth in popularity of video conferencing, virtual reality and internet 'chat rooms' arises from people's ability to come together regardless of physical distance from the organizing venue. Thus, as the concept of distance is less tied to physical geography, the rate and speed of certain social interactions and their consequences are being altered.

Our most immediate sense of the changing timeframe of social interaction in the globalizing world around us is that of increasing speed. To a certain extent, any social change generates certain feelings of nostalgia. Like the small town portrayed in the Frank Capra film, *It's a Wonderful Life*, successive generations can feel a sense of 'times past' when the pace of life was slower and seemingly more compatible with family and community life. Beyond nostalgia, life has objectively speeded up because of technological advances. In the workplace, the adoption of factory production lines, principles of 'scientific management' (Taylor 1911), and ever faster office machinery, such as the photocopier, and computing, has reduced the time taken to do a wide range of tasks. In the home, many so-called 'time-saving devices' have become mass consumer items (washing machines, dishwashers, microwave ovens) to free us (mainly women) from the drudgery of housework. Today, Gleick (1999) describes the contemporary world as filling up with fast-food drive-through restaurants, multi-tasking, speed dialling, instant credit and other time-saving features. Along with the capacity to live faster are pressures driving us to do so. The lives of many have become dominated by a constant race against the clock, some of it self-imposed by ambition and aspiration, but much of it integral to the pace and structure of postmodern society.

The technological capacity to live life at breakneck speed has been the enabling force for this acceleration of timeframes. Advances in transportation and communication technologies, in particular, have allowed us to interact at a far greater pace and intensity than ever before. Before mechanized transport, contact among population groups was regulated by the physical distance that people could travel by foot or animal. Natural barriers such as mountains and large bodies of water imposed certain limits to the geographical extent of such travel. The harnessing of new forms of energy by various modes of transport has permitted greater numbers of people to travel longer distances at a faster pace. The advent of the steam engine, for example, was a key development during the Industrial Revolution, opening up vast territories to European settlement and the establishment of intercontinental communication systems (for example postal services, telegraphy). Mass transportation in the twentieth century, via the burning of fossil fuels and the combustion engine – the automobile, jet aircraft – meant ever more people on the move. The availability of cheap commercial flights, in particular, has allowed ever-increasing numbers to travel frequently and more rapidly about the world.

Developments in communication and information technologies have had an equally dramatic impact on the speed and frequency of social interaction. Historically, the effective governing of any society has been strongly reliant on communication systems. Large empires, such as the Roman Empire, were highly dependent on reliable means of information flow from the centre to the farthest territories and back again. During the Industrial Revolution, the invention of telegraphy, radio and telephony during the nineteenth century allowed commerce and trade to flourish, as well as to facilitate the European colonization of far-flung territories. During the twentieth century, wire-based (telephone, fax, cable television) and radiowave-based (television, satellites, mobile telephones) modes of communication developed rapidly, progressively increasing the speed and reducing the cost of long-distance communication. By the last two decades of the century, the widespread use of personal computers, digital technology and ever-higher capacity microprocessors[1] (Table 4.1) began to lead to a merging of different media such as the Integrated Services Digital Network (ISDN). Such technologies have come to permeate so many aspects of everyday life. For example, any economic activities that require the acquisition of information, such as decisions about investment options, comparison shopping or sourcing inputs, can be done far quicker through the internet than traditional postal services, printed material or telephone (Butler et al. 1997).

It is important to recognize, however, that the temporal dimension of global change is not only about ever-increasing speed. The increasing scale and complexity of societies in a global age is a major social challenge because of larger populations, their geographical dispersal, and denser social networks among individuals and institutions. For example, members of a community have traditionally been defined by such factors as family name, birthplace, ethnicity or religion. Modern technologies enable us to become members of other types of communities, defined for instance by class, profession, gender, medical condition, political ideology or other special interest, that we can readily

Table 4.1   Developments in processing speeds of computers

Date	Computer processor	Average speed	Average price
1981	Intel 8086	4.77 MHz	US$5000
1982	Intel 80286	20 MHz	US$5000
1985	Intel 80386	40 MHz	US$5000
1989	Intel 80486	66 MHz	US$4000
1993	Pentium	166 MHz	US$3000
1995	Pentium Pro	200 MHz	US$3000
1997	Pentium II	450 MHz	US$3000
1998	Pentium III	1000 MHz	US$2000
2001	Pentium IV	2200+ MHz	US$2000

Source: Compiled from R. DeGrandpre (1999), *Ritalin Nation, Rapid-Fire Culture and the Transformation of Human Consciousness* (New York: W. W. Norton), p. 29; and Intel (2002), 'Processor Hall of Fame', <www.intel.com>

interact with across time and space. The proliferation of specialist web-sites and electronic 'listserves' embodies this proliferation of new 'virtual communities'. Depending on the intensity of the social interaction, members are bound together by shared goals, exchange of information and mutual support.

Our ability to wear multiple 'hats', however, can be restricted by our capacity to sufficiently sustain so many social identities. Being 'spread too thin' so that we have insufficient time to devote 'quality time' to each social identity is a common experience. Research on child development finds that parent–child relationships demand a certain amount of 'quality time' for healthy relationships to form. For instance, a study by Carlson et al. (1995) concludes that the imposition of a parent's timeframe on their baby's activities, rather than parental adaptation to the baby's pace, predicts distractability as an early precursor of later hyperactivity in middle childhood. Similarly, Whitelegg (1993) cites a novel by Michael Ende entitled *Momo* (1984) which depicts a small community persuaded by 'time thieves' to stop wasting time on idle conversations, care of the elderly and other communal activities. The result is not more available time but the mysterious vanishing of time: 'no matter how much time he saved, he never had any to spare; in some mysterious way, it simply vanished. Imperceptibly at first, but then quite unmistakably, his days grew shorter and shorter.' The novel refers to the breakdown of community as a result of our hurried lives, and the need for a greater investment of time to maintain appropriate relationships with families and friends. Whitelegg coins the concept of 'social speed' to describe the paradox that people feel they have *less* time despite the availability of faster modes of transport. This is because we use speed to travel further and more often, rather than saving time to spend elsewhere. Hence, we end up spending the same amount of time travelling overall, and perhaps even more, as congestion becomes a problem.

There are also aspects of human cognition that are resistant to time pressures. The greater availability of information, for instance, is not met by an equivalent capacity of the human brain to absorb and process this information. Faced with too much information, we experience 'information overload' which can slow our ability to act. This may be especially so in the health field. Health-related activities are the second most common use of the Internet, mostly by patients seeking information on conditions relevant to them. Indeed, health is a knowledge-intense industry, with doctors in the UK spending almost as long dealing with information (25 per cent of their time) as they do patient contact (Lister 2000: 182). Coiera (1996: 3) points to a potential problem in 'the mismatch in the speed with which new scientific results can be disseminated and the length of time required for careful peer review'. Similarly, the increased size and complexity of organizations of global reach can mean a slowing down of decision making and action. The term 'bureaucracy' in the late twentieth century has come to be synonymous with ponderousness, a reflection of the inverse relationship that can develop between the size of an organization and its capacity to act quickly.

Hence, there are dual forces impacting on our perception and experience of time amid globalization. In many ways, the technological capacity to live life in the 'fast lane' has led to social and cultural changes to our aspirations and lifestyles. In other ways, we are resistant to such pressures biologically, culturally and socially. Initially perhaps, it might be argued that the hyperactive, caffeine-addicted lifestyles of the so-called 'Type A personality' are limited to the world of big business and high finance of the industrialized world. In his study of the pace of life in different cultures, Levine (1997) argues that the concept of time is culture-specific. Switzerland, Ireland, Germany and Japan are judged as having the fastest pace of life,[2] Mexico, Indonesia and Brazil the slowest. It is argued here, however, that globalization is spreading the culture of speed to other countries, social classes and population groups. The result is that more and more of us feel like Charlie Chaplin in the 1936 film *Modern Times*, disoriented about the purpose of all of this frenetic modernity. For human health, there is a diverse range of consequences.

4.3   The global spectre of infectious disease: the quick and the dead

Moving such an infection across the Atlantic in the early sixteenth century must have involved a certain measure of chance, for the voyage was generally longer than a month, the average length of an active smallpox infection. Unless the passage were unusually fast, more than one previously unexposed person would have to be on board for the disease to be sustained across the Atlantic and thus passed to the Americans.

(Hays, 1998: 75)

The increase in international air travel, trade, and tourism will dramatically increase the prospects that infectious disease pathogens such as influenza – and vectors such as mosquitoes and rodents – will spread quickly around the globe, often in less time than the incubation period of most diseases.

U.S. National Intelligence Council, *The Global Infectious Disease Threat and Its Implications for the US* (2000)

Time is central to the spread of infections. All infectious agents must spread to new hosts at a certain rate to reproduce. The course of an epidemic, for example, depends on the rate of contact between susceptible and infectious individuals. In the field of mathematical epidemiology, this is known as the 'mass action principle' which holds that 'the net rate of spread of infection is assumed to be proportional to the product of the density of susceptible people times the density of infectious individuals' (Anderson and May 1991). Also important is the interplay between the individual and the social/natural environment, along with the nature of the viral or bacterial agent itself. Some infections, such as influenza and measles, need to pass quickly to new populations or die out. In other cases, such as variant Creutzfeldt-Jakob disease (vCJD) and HIV/AIDS, there is a long incubation period before illness appears, during which the virus can be passed on to others. Still others have an ability to survive for long periods outside of living tissue (e.g. anthrax) or in animal reservoirs (e.g. plague). The complex interaction between infection and environment is well illustrated by cholera. Classical *Vibrio cholerae*, the strain of cholera of the great pandemics of the nineteenth century, was gradually replaced by the milder El Tor strain during the twentieth century. The former could kill within days, and even hours, from severe dehydration. As water and sanitation systems improved in Europe, such a rapid rate of mortality did not allow sufficient time for the organism to spread and infect others. El Tor cholera produced a milder and longer illness, as well as a higher number of asymptomatic cases. This enabled it to become the dominant form of cholera throughout the world (Lee 2001b).

The potential impact of globalization on the epidemiology of infectious diseases has been the subject of much high-level attention. From the late nineteenth century, improvements in sanitation, water supplies, nutrition and housing in many industrialized countries, along with advances in health care such as the availability of antibiotics and vaccines, led to a remarkable decline in infectious diseases such as tuberculosis, cholera, typhoid and smallpox. Life expectancy at birth increased from 25–30 years in 1700 to 70–75 years by 1970, largely achieved by a decline in deaths from directly transmittable viral and bacterial infections (Anderson and May 1991: 3). While infectious diseases continue to afflict many in the developing world, those living in high-income countries came to feel relatively safe and even complacent. Much was made of the 'demographic–epidemiological transition' defined as 'the process by which falling fertility and mortality produce markedly rapid declines in communicable disease among the young, leading to ageing populations with a rising proportion of older members among whom chronic disorders predominate' (Gwatkin et al. 1999). It was assumed to be only a matter of time before economic development, and thus the benefits of modern health care, would spread to poor countries.

Yet, even as the global eradication of smallpox was being celebrated in the late 1970s, an unprecedented achievement of medical science and international cooperation, dark clouds were on the horizon. Malaria, the target of eradication efforts for decades, was proving a resilient and even growing problem. Tuberculosis, quietly forgotten despite killing around one million people annually (primarily in the developing world), was declared a 'global emergency' by WHO in 1993. Twenty diseases that had been in decline have re-emerged or spread geographically between 1973 and 1999 including multi-drug-resistant forms of TB, malaria and cholera. And new challenges loomed. Twenty-nine new diseases were identified during the same period, of which HIV/AIDS is perhaps the most prominent. Worldwide infectious diseases are a leading cause of death, accounting for up to one-third of all deaths in 1998. By 2001, total deaths to date from AIDS surpassed 20 million (UNAIDS 2001a), thus exceeding deaths from the bubonic plague during the Middle Ages and influenza in 1918–19 (estimated 20 million each). Even in a wealthy country like the United States, there has been a doubling of deaths from infectious diseases since the late 1990s (US National Intelligence Council 2000).

These developments have shaken the confidence of the health community, and complacency has been replaced by fears that contagion is back with a vengeance. The element of time is central to these contemporary fears about the resurgence of infectious disease. As well as the changing spatial distribution of disease, there is growing evidence that current forms of globalization provide fertile conditions for the more rapid spread of certain infections. The movement of people via modern transportation systems, rapid urbanization without adequate water, sanitation and public health facilities, human-induced environmental changes (see Chapter 3), and the intensified exchange of goods and services may be contributing to the increased speed with which infectious agents can arise and spread worldwide. A new sense of vulnerability to infectious diseases, in short, has accompanied the present era of accelerating globalization (Kassalow 2001; Barks-Ruggles 2001). In this context, lethal diseases that are fastest to spread have captured popular imaginations. The dreaded Ebola virus has become mythologized as embodying the worst of nightmares among infectious diseases – the quick and the deadly.

The increase and spread of antimicrobial resistance (AMR) is another example of the importance of the temporal dimension of globalization to infectious disease. There are several links between globalization and growing AMR that require further study. Current evidence suggests that the overuse and misuse of antimicrobials, for human and veterinary use (such as for intensive rearing of animals for food production) are the key factors. By the 1970s more than 100 antibiotics were available but extensive misuse has one by one led to resistance. It is estimated that 20–50 per cent of the 145 million prescriptions given each year to outpatients in high-income countries are unnecessary (Stolberg 1998: 45), and up to 75 per cent of antibiotic use is of questionable therapeutic value (Wise et al. 1998: 609). Seventy per cent of all antibiotics are used for growth promoters in livestock. The above, coupled with the decline in public health systems that ensure appropriate use of such drugs, have directly contributed to the emergence of so-called 'superbugs'. These are microbes that are resistant to one or more of the arsenal of drugs that medical practitioners have come to rely on since the introduction of penicillin in 1943, to treat bacterial infections. The list of drug-resistant microbes grows steadily – *Streptococcus pneumoniae*, *Mycobacterium tuberculosis*, *Neisseria gonorrhoeae* and, perhaps most worryingly, methicillin resistant *Staphylococcus aureas* (MRSA) and

Vancomycin Intermediate-Resistant *Staphylococcus aureas* (VISA). More than 90 per cent of *Staphylococcus aureas* strains are now resistant to penicillin and a wide range of other antibiotics including methicillin, considered the penultimate line of defence before vancomycin.

The potential for these 'superbugs' to spread worldwide in a short time is already known. As Alexander Tomasz, Chief of Microbiology at Rockefeller University (as quoted in Stolberg 1998: 45), warns, 'These are international problems. The next wave of bugs is just a few days away.' For instance, a multidrug resistant strain of *Streptococcus pneumoniae* originating in Spain spread throughout the world in a matter of weeks during the early 1990s (US National Intelligence Council 2000: 10). The first case of VISA was detected in Japan in December 1996, and was followed by cases in the US from 1998 onwards. AMR has thus led to an intense race to develop new drugs before the effectiveness of existing ones, notably vancomycin, is undermined. A new generation of antimicrobials will take several years to develop and, if not achieved faster than the development and spread of AMR (bacteria divide once every twenty minutes), will mean a return to the pre-penicillin era when familiar infections could become fatal, routine surgery could become high risk, and new microbes could spread unchecked.

By their very nature, therefore, infectious diseases evoke within us an almost primeval fear, intensified by the prospect that globalization will 'level the playing field' in terms of susceptibility once again. While humanitarian concerns toward the afflictions of the developing world remain, there has been a certain degree of over-confidence that diseases such as TB, cholera and malaria remain 'over there'. Globalization changes this. Equally important, however, is the prospect that conditions in high-income countries are also leading to the emergence of new infections and threatening our ability to effectively treat infections through antimicrobials. In this sense, responsibility for addressing the changing nature of infectious diseases is global.

4.4   Fast food and slow death: diet and nutrition in a world hooked on speed

Prepared, precooked, prepackaged meals – all the descendants of the TV Dinner – now take up more supermarket space than fresh fruits and vegetables. They threaten to surpass the rest of the traditional stock: the mere ingredients of meals.

James Gleick, *Faster, the Acceleration of Just About Everything* (1999)

The reunification of Germany took place on October 3rd, 1990 ... Two months later, eastern Germany had its first McDonalds.

Eric Schlosser, *Fast-Food Nation* (2002)

In traditional societies, food production and consumption occupy a substantial proportion of daily life. The industrialization of food has dramatically changed our relationship with food over time with trends towards larger economies of scale, mass production, highly specialized supply chains, widespread mechanization and the use of a variety of processing methods to add value. All of these changes have contributed to a reduction in time needed by most people to meet this basic human need. Yet these changes have important implications for our health.

On the production side, there has been a wide range of developments to meet the dual pressures of increasing demand for food by growing populations, and reducing costs in an increasingly competitive global market. Producers have sought greater yields through more intense farming methods such as battery farms for chickens, feedlots for cattle, and monocropping of single species and/or varieties of plants. This has been accompanied by selective breeding to produce fast-growing animals and plants with desirable qualities, and the increased use of fertilizers, antibiotics, growth hormones and increasingly genetic modification to speed production. The result has been a remarkable change in the rate of food production. Engel (2001a) notes, for example, that twenty years ago, broiler chickens were raised in 84 days. Today they are ready for slaughter in half the time. This has been achieved through selective breeding of chickens capable of turning feed into flesh quickly. Up to the 1940s, more than 90 per cent of American cattle were grass-fed, roaming cattle ranches and eating native grasses or hay. Grass-fed beef then needed to be hung for a few weeks before being sold and consumed. From the 1950s, cattle began to be penned into feedlots, fed cheap grains and later processed plant and animal by-products, and sold for consumption days after slaughter. Following such practices, the US company Monfort Inc. expanded its annual production capacity from 20,000 head of cattle in the 1940s to almost one million cattle per year today (Schlosser 2002)

As well as increasing yields, producers have added value to basic food products through greater processing. There are now at least 3000 different additives used in food processing, ranging from sugar and salt to artificial colours and preservatives. Additives are used for four main reasons: to enhance the appeal of foods; to improve nutritional value;

to facilitate processing (including stabilizers, thickeners); and to preserve freshness and prevent spoilage. The latter includes food irradiation, a method used to extend the shelf life of perishable foods (for example long-life milk) and thus increase their marketability.

Accompanying developments in food production have been corresponding changes in patterns of food consumption. In populations around the world, there is a clear trend towards food that takes less time to prepare and consume. High 'time intensity' staple dishes, even in low-income countries, are giving way to 'the selection of foods that require less time and skill to prepare and consume' (Drewnoski and Popkin 1997: 37). In the US, where changes in food practices are most prominent, three-quarters of meals a generation ago were made at home. Today, most meals are prepared outside of the home, mainly at fast-food restaurants. Roughly one-quarter of Americans buy fast foods each day. Between 1960 and 1997, the amount of ready chips that the average American ate increased from three and a half pounds each year to 30 pounds per year (Schlosser 2002). Along with highly processed foods, there has been a greater use of microwave ovens to cook and reheat food in a fraction of the time of convection ovens. Other inventions include foods that 'boil in a bag', toast and cook instantly by adding hot water.

There are a variety of reasons for the popularity of 'convenience' foods – the rise in the number of women in the workforce, gradual adaptation of palates to processed foods and, not least, the intense marketing of such products (see Chapter 5). Speeding the time needed for food production and consumption offers tangible benefits. There are clear pressures in some countries to increase yields to meet the needs of growing populations. The ability to store food for longer periods, without the risk of deterioration or contamination by harmful microorganisms, has been a major contribution of modern food production methods. Up to one-half of the world's food supply is lost after harvesting as a result of spoilage, infestation, and bacterial and fungal attack (Craft 1994). Methods such as canning, drying, freezing, pasteurization, heat treatment, use of preservatives and irradiation have extended the 'shelf life' of many foods. The risks from foodborne diseases are serious. Up to 70 per cent of diarrhoeal diseases, which cause about a quarter of all deaths in low-income countries, are due to infected food. The preservation of food also enables it to be consumed at different times of the year, or to be traded more widely, enabling a diversification of the nutritional content of human diets.

However, the adverse effects of the industrialization of food are also increasingly recognized. As described in Chapter 3, the globalization of the food industry has placed a strong emphasis on economies of scale and mass production, sometimes at the expense of quality, the environment and biodiversity. Furthermore, there are close links between the way food is produced and our health. One major concern is the rising incidence of obesity in many industrialized countries, and among the relatively affluent populations of middle and low-income countries. As a result of what Lang (1999b) calls the 'burgerization' of our diets, coupled with more sedentary lifestyles, the number of obese and overweight people has dramatically risen. The people of most high-income countries have been getting bigger, both in height and weight, over several centuries. Between 1750 and 1950, average British male heights increased by about 20 centimetres, and working-class 14-year-old boys by 31 centimetres (Appleby 1997). In Scandinavian countries, for example, the average increment is about 1.5 centimetres per generation (20 years) or 7.5 centimetres per century. This earlier growth is largely attributable to improvements in nutrition, such as postwar milk consumption, and predates the advent of fast food (Boseley 2001b). The size-gains in recent decades, however, need to be seen in a different light. While gains in average height are slowing, rapid increases in average weight have continued. During the 1990s, the prevalence of overweight adults increased by 50 per cent in the US (Strauss et al. 2001), with most US adults (56.4 per cent) being overweight (Mokdad et al. 2001). The number of obese adults[3] increased by 61 per cent between 1991 and 2000, accounting for one in five adults (Mokdad et al. 2001). Half of Europeans and 61 per cent of Americans are now overweight (Josefson 2001). Worryingly, similar trends are being observed among younger people (13–18-year-olds) and children (4–12-year-olds). Targeted by the marketing of fast food, these two cohorts are now described as undergoing an epidemic of obesity in the US, Europe and other high-income countries (Dietz 1998). Among American children, between 1986 and 1998 overweight prevalence increased by more than 120 per cent among African Americans and Hispanics, and 50 per cent among whites. By 1998, 21.5 per cent of African American, 21.8 per cent of Hispanic and 12.3 per cent of white children were overweight (Strauss and Pollack 2001).

Despite variations in definition and measurement, making it impossible to give an overview of the global prevalence of obesity, studies worldwide consistently report high prevalence and increasing rates in other countries (Frühbeck 2000; WHO 1997a). In a growing number of low and middle-income countries, these trends are most notable among the relatively affluent that can afford, and have chosen, to adopt Western diets and lifestyles (WHO 2001a). As markets in the developed world are saturated, fast food companies expand abroad, using the appeal of 'Americana and the promise of modernization' (Schlosser 2002) to attract new consumers, notably young children aged two to eight. Just as working-class parents during the 1950s aspired to eating in restaurants, people in the developing world accord themselves a certain status and self-esteem by eating in fast-food restaurants. The so-called 'nutrition transition' by which western diets are being adopted in lower and middle-income countries (Popkin 1994) is underpinned by a cognitive transition.

The health consequences of excess weight are well documented. There are an estimated 300,000 deaths from obesity-related diseases in the US annually, second only to tobacco (Allison et al. 1999). Coronary heart disease, gallbladder disease, colorectal cancer, metabolic diseases, infertility, hypoventilation, arrhythmia, raised blood pressure, sleep apnoea and depression are all associated with being overweight. For people with a body mass index above 35 (obese), there is a 93-fold increase in risk for women and 43-fold increase for men of diabetes mellitis. Obesity is an important determinant of cardiovascular disease (CVD), notably as a consequence of hypertension, and a major contributor in the 33 per cent rise in diagnosed diabetes between 1990 and 1998 (Mokdad et al. 2000a), accounting for up to 10 per cent of US adults. It is clear that genes related to obesity are not responsible because the US gene pool did not change significantly during this period (Mokdad et al. 2000b). Children that grow quickly during the first three years of life (higher-than-average increase in BMI), because they are allowed to eat as much as they want, are more at risk of becoming diabetic during childhood. Childhood type 1 diabetes is becoming more common in affluent countries because of the abundance of food. In Britain, the incidence of child diabetes has doubled in the past five years, with 1200 children diagnosed each year (EURODIAB ACE Study Group 2000). Worldwide, diabetes mellitus affects 100 million people and accounts for 8 per cent of total health budgets in high-income countries (WHO 1996a).

There are other health concerns raised by changes in food production and consumption patterns. There is growing evidence, marked by high-profile outbreaks, that the ways in which food production methods have changed have also contributed to the increased spread of foodborne diseases such as *Salmonella* serotype *enteritidis* (SE),

ınd vCJD (Lee and Patel 2002). For example, the intense
ls, accompanied by high speed and volume production
.....ouses, raises the risk of contamination (Schlosser 2002).
ı nese risks, in turn, can be rapidly dispersed through the global food trade. Farm imports into the US increased 65 per cent between 1991 and 1999 (Barks-Ruggles 2001). Other concerns have been raised over the potential link between the greater use of additives in processed foods and the increased incidence of hyperactivity (see below) and allergies in children. There are also disputed concerns over the safety of microwave ovens and food irradiation (Public Citizen 2000).

In summary, changes to how food is produced and consumed has been part of the acceleration of lifestyles, and the globalization of such lifestyles. Food is now a global industry, one that shapes the quality of the food available to us and the ways we consume it. Given real and perceived constraints on our time, our focus is increasingly on speed. As well as losing the social benefits of preparing and eating meals communally, the eating habits of modern societies are creating serious health risks far beyond indigestion.

4.5   The mental health effects of temporal change

> *… both the pace of life and the intensity of the stimulus world around us continue to intensify, largely because of ongoing transformations taking place in the modes of human experience … As they do, they're also radically transforming time, space, and the fabric of human consciousness. Rapid-fire culture gives rise to rapid-fire consciousness, an unsettling temporal disturbance of the self that then motivates an escape from slowness …*

Richard DeGrandpre, Ritalin Nation (1999:22)

There are growing signs that the accelerating pace of life is having adverse impacts on mental health. Historically, mental health has been the Cinderella of public health practice. Yet about 500 million people worldwide suffer from mental disorders, and the trend is upwards. The total burden of disease from mental illness is expected to grow from 12 per cent in 2001 to 15 per cent in 2020. Mental disorders represent four of the ten leading causes of disability worldwide, with depressive disorders due to rise from the fourth to second leading cause of death and disability (WHO 2001: 3). An analysis of studies on major depression from North America, Western Europe, Middle East, Asia and the Pacific Rim finds the condition increasing over time and occurring

earlier for successively younger age cohorts in many different locations. The age of onset of manic depression has declined from 32 years
in the mid 1960s to 19 years by the late 1990s (Cross-National
Collaborative Group 1992).

WHO cites three main factors behind these trends – increased
poverty, ageing populations, and the pace of modern living. As WHO
Director-General Gro Harlem Brundtland (2001a) describes,

> We are living in a world of rapid change. This is experienced by
> people living in the calmest and most prosperous corners of the
> world. They encounter newness at a breath-taking pace: from
> new technology to new jobs to new fashions in entertainment
> and culture. They are being swirled along in the rapidity of global
> transformation.

The most commonly cited mental health manifestation of such rapid
change is stress. As Bonn and Bonn (2000) write, '[s]tress, in essence, is
a feeling of doubt about being able to cope, a perception that the
resources available do not match the demands made. When it persists,
stress can cause physical and psychological ill-health and adversely
affect social functioning.' In the work environment, stress levels are
linked to how much control one has over work demands. The less
latitude that an individual has over decisions affecting workload, the
higher the level of stress.

The lack of control over the pace and nature of work as a result of
globalization is an important factor in growing rates of mental illness.
The changes taking place are partly the result of economic restructuring as large companies move their operations to find cheaper work-
forces, 'downsize' or replace workers with technology, and enforce
'more flexible' terms of work to ensure global competitiveness.
Agricultural workers may face greater insecurity of livelihood given
declining terms of trade, more expensive seeds and other inputs, and
domination of the sector by global companies. Even in countries such
as China and Japan, where the 'iron rice bowl' was a traditional symbol
of economic and social stability, there are now few 'jobs for life'. Thus,
workers fortunate to have gainful employment must work harder than
ever to maintain job security. With few exceptions, people in high-
income countries are working longer hours, spurred by insecurities in
the job market (Cooper 2001). The unemployed and underemployed
face the mental stress of lack of work and possible impoverishment. As
Brundtland (2001a) writes, 'people exposed to rapid change have to

cope with insecurity and unpredictability. And, some of the consequences of change clearly are negative. This is especially the case if
change is imposed on people who are powerless to influence how it
affects them.'

The manifestations of work-related stress are increasing levels of
sleep disturbance, gastric and duodenal ulcers, dyspepsia and irritable
bowel syndrome. One of the biggest selling drugs in the world is
Zantac®, a treatment for peptic ulcers. Work stress is also associated
with cardiovascular risk factors such as hypertension and hypercholes-
terolaemia. When first diagnosed in the 1980s, it was argued that
chronic fatigue syndrome (CFS) might be a result of 'burn out' or
depression by high-flying workers. The high prevalence among young
professional women, in particular, led to the condition being dubbed
the 'yuppie flu'. While many health professionals now recognize it as a
physical, rather than mental, illness, the cause remains unknown and
effective treatment includes the use of anti-depressants and cognitive
behavioural therapy (Reid et al. 2000).

Another manifestation of our heightened desire for speed and urgency
in modern society is the rising incidence of 'road rage'. Road rage is
defined as a driver reacting with anger at another driver, with the anger
overtly expressed and communicated. Others use the term 'aggressive
driving incidents' which are defined as events in which an angry or impa-
tient driver tries to injure or kill another driver after a traffic dispute. As
individuals seek to travel by car more frequently and, in many cases,
more quickly, traffic congestion[4] or other obstructions cause heightened
frustration. The US National Highway Traffic Safety Administration
(NHTSA) estimates that 66 per cent of road traffic fatalities in the US (up
to 1200 people) are caused by aggressive driving behaviours such as
passing on the right (left hand drive), running red lights and tailgating.
Such events have increased by 51 per cent since 1990, with 37 per cent of
incidents involving firearms (Mizell 1996). Studies in the UK, Canada and
Australia show similar trends (Joint 1995). As well as the environmental
impact, it is believed that the spread of the automobile culture to other
parts of the world is creating similar experiences.

A further example is the controversy over attention deficit hyperactivity disorder (ADHD). Variations in definition, benchmarks in diagnosis, and even nonrecognition of the condition in some countries
make accurate global prevalence data impossible. Nonetheless, it is
increasingly recognized that ADHD is a common but complex condition characterized by excessive inattentiveness, impulsiveness or
hyperactivity that significantly interferes with everyday life. What is

disputed is the cause of this condition and its appropriate treatment. Many medical professionals hold that it is a genetically inherited condition of brain dysfunction as shown in cerebral imaging studies. If accurately diagnosed, multidisciplinary management including treatment with drugs such as methylphenidate (Ritalin) is found to be highly effective. If untreated, the disorder may interfere with educational and social development, and predispose to psychiatric and other difficulties (Kewley 1998).

Others, however, question the medicalization of ADHD. In his book, *Ritalin Nation*, DeGrandpre (1999) questions why ADHD has become the most commonly diagnosed child psychiatric disorder in the US, with Ritalin prescribed in 90 per cent of the cases. Prior to the 1960s, hyperactivity was rarely treated as a medical problem. In 1961 the US Food and Drug Administration (FDA) approved Ritalin for use in children with behavioural problems. He writes that by 1975, 150,000 children were being prescribed drugs to reduce hyperactivity. This rose to about a million American children by the late 1980s, and two million by the late 1990s. It is now estimated that ADHD affects 7 per cent of US children between 6 and 11 years (CDC 2002). The US consumes 80–90 per cent of Ritalin in the world. DeGrandpre asks whether this increase in ADHD is a reaction to the faster pace of modern life and, in particular, overstimulation received by children. He and others (Armstrong 1995; Hallowell and Ratey 1995) cite the pressures of time and availability of constant, fast-paced stimuli in everyday life as contributing to the creation of 'restless minds and impulsive personalities'. He argues, 'the speedup of culture means we experience more stimulus events each day, but the nature of these events also has undergone a dramatic transformation' (DeGrandpre 1999:27). The result is children unable to focus attention on 'slow' activities such as schoolwork, instead craving constant stimulation through computer games, television and other intense experiences.

Is attention deficit disorder (ADD or as it is now called, attention deficit hyperactivity disorder, or ADHD) really a newly discovered medical disease, or is it a culture-induced brain dysfunction that results from our growing addiction to speed? Might the craze over stimulants like cocaine, crack, methamphetamine, and ecstasy in the 1980s and 1990s have a deep cultural connection to our speeding-up society? And might the rush for speed also be connected with the rise of coffee/caffeine culture and the Ritalin solution? (DeGrandpre 1999:16)

While evidence of the above trends in mental health come largely from the US, where fast-paced lifestyles are most pronounced, the export of these lifestyles through processes of globalization raise the prospect of similar experiences in other countries and population groups, notably those most 'plugged into' the globalization lifestyle. Norman Sartorious, head of the European Association of Psychiatrists (as quoted in Holden 2000: 39), argues that depression is often thought of as a by-product of high-stress, urban and western lifestyles, but it is worsening in low-income countries. Greater economic insecurity, the physical effects of malnutrition and infections, war and social dislocation may all be contributing to a future epidemic of mental health. As Lewis Judd, former chief of the US National Institute of Mental Health (NIH) puts it, 'I see depression as the plague of the modern era' (as cited in Holden 2000: 40).

4.6　Designer genes: Evolution out of the window?

Sequencing the human genome is one of the transforming events in science – events that change our whole view of where we stand in the universe. Ever since Darwin we've been trying to understand the detail of how the world got to be the way it is, but it's only now that we are beginning to understand the history of life as it's written in our genes.

Sir Robert May, Chief Adviser to the UK Government (2000)

The evolutionary process, according to Darwinian theory, occurs at the speed at which ecological pressure is exerted, and an adaptive response through natural selection is elicited. Depending on the life cycle of the organism in question, evolution can occur in a few minutes (as with bacteria) or over hundreds of years (e.g. oak trees). Importantly, evolution occurs synchronically with other organisms and the natural environment. The process is a continuously dynamic yet gradual one of adaptation and response.

The advent of increasingly sophisticated methods of genetic modification, whereby genetic material (Box 4.1) is selected, removed or manipulated to strengthen or weaken particular characteristics of an organism, creates the capacity to alter the timescale of natural evolution. The manipulation of genetic material is, of course, far from new. Agricultural practices dating back 10,000 years or so sought to give Mother Nature a helping hand through selective breeding of plants and animals. Indeed, defenders of the current use of genetically modified organisms (GMOs) argue that the technology is simply an extension of such practices. However, it is important to distinguish among three methods of genetic modification: (a) crossbreeding of different individuals of the same species (undertaken for at least 10,000 years); (b) crossing sexually incompatible species of the same genus (since the 1970s); and (c) moving specific segments of genetic material between unrelated organisms (since the early 1980s). What is distinct today is the widespread use of the latter two methods, potentially resulting in more far reaching changes to the genetic makeup of plants and animals, and at an unprecedented rate of change. This has a range of implications for human health.

The question of timeframe is central to debates about GMOs. In nature, plants and animals battle it out for survival and dominance,

---

Box 4.1   What's in a gene?

The field of genetics is the study of heredity and variation in individuals and the means whereby characteristics are passed from parent to offspring. The founder of genetic research was Gregor Mendel, an Austrian monk, who studied the passing of genetic information between yellow and green garden peas during the early nineteenth century. The field developed rapidly from the early twentieth century into many subfields, such as population genetics and molecular genetics, and later becoming entangled in political ideology (eugenics).

The gene is the fundamental unit of genetic material found at a specific location on a chromosome. There are 24 chromosomes in the human body. A gene, of which there are around 30,000–40,000 in humans of varying size, is chemically complex. The genetic code refers to the specific information, carried by DNA (deoxyribonucleic acid) molecules, that control the particular amino acids and their positions in every protein, and thus all the proteins synthesized within a cell. The shape of a DNA molecule is the double helix. DNA information is coded into nucleotides (or bases) of four types: A, G, C and T for short. A change in the genetic code results in an amino acid being inserted incorrectly in a protein resulting in a mutation. Genetic engineering (recombinant DNA technology) is the artificial modification of an organisms's genetic make-up.

There are various types of genes depending on their function. Genes can be dominant, with the characteristic occurring whenever the gene is present, or recessive, with the characteristic occurring only when the gene is present in both members of the chromosome pair (homozygous). The total information stored in the chromosomes of an organism is known as its genome.

Sources: US Department of Energy (1992), *Primer on Molecular Genetics* (Washington DC: DOE Human Genome Program); and Jones S., *In the Blood: God, Genes and Destiny* (London: Flamingo, 1997).

with evolutionary competition taking place gradually and continually over generations. At this pace, other organisms adapt simultaneously so that the entirety of the natural world is in constant and interdependent flux. The use of modern methods of genetic modification introduces changes within a single generation, allowing certain genes to dominate according to selected criteria. The food industry, for example, uses these techniques to breed for characteristics that improve profitability such as disease and pest resistance, frost tolerance, herbicide tolerance and ripening delay (Beringer 1999). These characteristics may or may not be compatible with those that would develop with natural evolution.

In many cases, tampering with evolution can yield beneficial results. Genetic engineering can speed the effectiveness of a baculovirus, a type of virus that infects caterpillars of certain moths, so that it kills pests before they have time to strip a tree of its foliage (Bishop et al. 1988). Research is also under way to develop and spread a synthetic gene throughout populations of the mosquito species that are vectors for human forms of malaria. Malaria infects 500 million people and causes two million deaths each year. As Meek (2001: 3) describes,

> Until now, spreading genes throughout a species was something only evolution was capable of, over millions of years of natural selection … [This research aims] to transform the malaria-carrying mosquito into a subtly different species – still a bloodsucking nuisance, but no longer a killer – within two to 25 years of releasing the first GM insects.

Genetic research on plants also holds much promise. The development of faster growing crops, such as varieties of rice that mature 30–50 days earlier and have 50 per cent higher yields, will produce much-needed food for growing populations. Other 'first generation' products have specific agronomic traits, including herbicide tolerance and insect resistance, to improve productivity. A further area of development is plant-based vaccines and other medically-related compounds (Dunwell 1999).

Current evidence suggests that consuming GMOs does not pose a direct health risk. Indeed, so-called 'second generation' products of GM foods, expected to reach consumer markets by 2020, will seek to improve product quality or higher value traits including added vitamins and micronutrients, modified starch and oil content, reduced levels of allergens and toxins, and resistance to freezing. However, there is some evidence that disrupting the intricate dance of evolution could have unforeseen and potentially irreversible consequences. Foremost are the potential environmental impacts. There are concerns that GMOs have already been extensively introduced without sufficient understanding of the long-term consequences for native and natural species of plants and animals. Over one-half of the soybean crop in the US is GMOs (Beringer 1999). The total world acreage of herbicide-tolerant and insect-protected corn, soybeans and cotton grew from 4 million to 102 million acres between 1996 and 2000, with estimates of potential global growth of up to 875 million acres (Monsanto 2000a:7). GM crops were grown in thirteen countries by 2001 and tested in dozens of others (Vidal and Aglionby 2001). Food products (for example soft drinks, salads, breads) containing GMOs are widely sold, generally without being labelled as such.

Claims that GMOs can be kept wholly separate from the natural environment are seen as foolhardy by some critics. There are numerous precedents of intentional and unintentional release or escape of plant and animal species into non-native environments, with direct consequences for indigenous species. At best, introduced species can become an interesting ecological anomaly, such as parakeets in the UK. In some cases, they can become unwanted pests that may cause damage to local habitats (e.g. rabbits and wild pigs in Australia). One-half of weed species in the US are nonindigenous plants (Pimentel 1986). In other cases, non-native species (e.g. ruddy duck and grey squirrel in the UK) can displace indigenous species and even cause them to become extinct. Furthermore, the global migration of plant diseases remains a serious concern. In May 2002, fears of a new disease called 'sudden oak death' caused by the fungus *Phytophthora ramorum* (the same family of fungus that caused the potato blight during the nineteenth century) led the UK government to ban plant imports under the Plant Health Act 1967 from parts of the US where the disease is rampant (Brown 2002b).

Despite industry reassurances, evidence of GMOs impacting on the natural environment has raised widespread concern. Tests on the toxicity of pollen[5] from GM maize for the monarch butterfly initially found the butterflies were harmed. However, the study fed the butterflies exclusively on food they would not normally eat, and with doses of pollen eight times the level likely to be found in the wild (Losey et al. 1999). Subsequent field research has found no significant differences between butterfly survival in areas planted with GM and conventional maize (Henderson 2000). GM maize has also been at the centre of findings by the Mexican government that, despite its own ban on GM maize, there are high levels (up to 95 per cent of samples) of contamination in areas that act as the gene bank for one of the world's staple crops. Mexico is home to hundreds of varieties of maize which are allowed to crossbreed in order to produce optimal crops for extreme conditions. It is suspected that corn imported from the US for food has been used by farmers as seed, unaware that it contains grain derived from GM crops. This conclusion is supported by the fact that the worst contamination was found near main roads where maize is sold to villagers. In remote areas, there was only 1–2 per cent contamination. It is unknown which variety of GM maize was responsible for the contamination because the three companies that produce the product, Monsanto, Syngenta and Aventis, use the same technology and refuse to disclose information on the protein used, on trade secrets grounds (Brown 2002).

A further health-related fear surrounding the widespread use of GMOs is the spread of genes from one microorganism to another by natural mechanisms, such as plasmids, raising the prospect that antibiotic resistance could be transferred to other species. Most GM products contain a gene for antibiotic resistance as a marker for scientists to spot which plants have taken on new genetic features. Research has found a wide range of genetic transfers between microorganisms living in various habitats including genes that confer antibiotic resistance. For example, resistance has been found to pass from *Enterobacteriaceae* living in the gut, to *Neisseria gonorrhoea*, the cause of venereal disease, and *Haemonphilus influenzae*, the cause of influenza, as a result of widespread use of antibiotics in modern medicine (Connor 1988).

The ultimate target of genetic modification, and perhaps the most controversial of all, is the human genome. When the Human Genome Project (HGP) completes its task (Box 4.2), namely mapping of the entire human genetic code, an entirely new world of R&D opens up. There is broad agreement that this information will yield positive benefits for human health. Medical applications are expected to revolutionize health care during the twenty-first century, enabling, for example, an improved ability to prevent or mitigate inherited disorders at an earlier stage. Other applications include the development of new drug therapies, treatments for addiction, and therapies for jet-lag and sleep disorders. At the same time, the 'genomic revolution' and the prospect of GM people raises a host of moral and ethical issues regarding the application of the technology. Early debate over ownership of the human genome has been resolved in favour of keeping it within the public domain, but not before a race by some biotechnology companies to obtain the code first in order to assert patent rights. There are also important issues concerning how knowledge about genetic makeup could be used, for example, in antenatal care, employment, immigration and the insurance industry.

Box 4.2   The Human Genome Project

The Human Genome Project is an international research programme initiated in 1986 involving scientists from 16 institutions in six countries (China, France, Germany, Japan, UK and US) to determine the DNA sequence of the entire human genetic code. The aim of the project is to determine the DNA sequence of the entire human genome which can then be used to identify an estimated, 30,000–40,000 genes, and to identify their positions on individual chromosomes. This entails a complete mapping of the genetic information contained in the chromosomes of the human species.

The project is funded by grants from government agencies and charitable trusts including a so-called 'peace dividend' from nuclear research by the US Department of Energy. The total cost of producing the complete sequence will be an estimated US$3 billion. In June 2000 the first working draft of the 'Book of Humankind' was completed and made publicly available. The final phase of the project, filling in gaps and increasing overall sequence accuracy, is due for completion in 2003.

It is believed that this information will transform health care in the twenty-first century by improving diagnosis and treatment of many inherited disorders such as cystic fibrosis and sickle cell anaemia, as well as other human illnesses such as cardiovascular disease, cancer and asthma. Genetic tests may eventually allow detection of predisposition to certain conditions, in turn, opening new avenues for preventive medicine. The development of more effective treatments may also be possible including the replacement of faulty genes with a correctly functioning one (gene therapy).

As well as the HGP, around twenty non-human organisms have been sequenced by scientists around the world. This research can provide clues to the functioning of human genes, and provide inexpensive models for studying different aspects of human genes such as cell division and growth of specialized tissue. The completed genomes so far include a number of disease-causing organisms of global significance including *Plasmodium falciparum* (malaria), *Mycobacterium tuberculosis* and methicillin-resistant *Staphylococcus aureus* (MRSA).

Source: International Human Genome Sequencing Consortium (2001), 'Initial sequencing and analysis of the human genome', *Nature*, 409, 13 February: 860–921; and US Department of Energy (1997), *Human Genome Program Report* (Washington DC: Office of Biological and Environmental Research).

Less deliberate than GM, yet far reaching, is the way in which intensifying population mobility is contributing to changes in the genetic makeup of human societies. In a world where people have become increasingly mobile, and one in a hundred people live in a country not of their birth, an unprecedented mingling of genetic pools is occurring known as genetic admixture. The greatest degree of genetic admixture can be found in countries with the highest rates of immigration such as the US, Canada and Australia.

The health consequences are mixed. On the positive side, greater genetic admixture can reduce the risk of inherited genetic disorders where both partners need to carry the relevant recessive gene. For instance, the high incidence of Tay-Sachs disease, a disorder of the central nervous system, among Ashkenazi Jews is due to the high proportion (one in eighteen) of carriers of the gene within the community compared to the US population as a whole (one in three hundred). Importantly, the strong cultural preference for marrying within the community has contributed to the higher incidence of the disease. By encouraging a greater mixing of genetic pools, genetic admixture reduces the statistical probability of such diseases being passed on to future generations.

On the more negative side, there is evidence that greater mobility of human genes can increase the risk of certain conditions. The presence of the sickle cell gene among Africans and their diaspora has been an evolutionary response to protect against malaria. Genetic admixture reduces this genetic resistance. It is also believed that one of the risk factors in pre-eclampsia, a potentially fatal condition in pregnancy, is the degree of genetic difference between the partners. The condition is caused by the rejection of the father's genetic material in the foetus by the mother's body, and interracial couples are thought to have an increased risk of this occurring (Ward and Lindheimer 1999). Beyond genetic admixture, the settlement of people of particular genetic makeup in a new social and natural environment may contribute to an increase in certain conditions. For example, South Asians settled around the world have higher rates of coronary heart disease (CHD), prevalence of non-insulin dependent diabetes (five times higher than Europeans), and hypertension than populations who have remained in the region. These patterns are not explainable by smoking prevalence or dietary features (for example percentage of energy from fat, ratio of polyunsaturates to saturates). Rather, these may all be manifestations of a single underlying syndrome, namely a result of past genetic adaptations to conditions of unreliable food supply and physically demanding work. As food supply becomes plentiful, and lifestyles change, South Asians may be more genetically prone to develop these conditions (McKeigue and Sevak 1994).

In summary, globalization is accelerating the movement of many kinds of genetic material around the world. As genomic research progresses, the desire to manipulate the links between genes and human welfare will increase. Human intervention in genetics, however, means enabling certain genes – some that may not otherwise do so – to dominate, and others not to. GM, for example, breaks down normal gene barriers through the insertion of genetic material from one species to another, and at a rate faster than nature would allow. The implications for the natural environment and human societies, and the complex ethical issues raised, are only beginning to be understood.

4.7   Environmental sustainability and global health

The accumulation of evidence has us extremely worried ... We have to get serious about global change. It is not only going to be a warmer world, it is going to be a sicker world.
Andrew Dobson, Princeton University as quoted in Radford (2002)

... there can be no trade and no economic development on a dead planet.
Edward Goldsmith, 'Global Trade and the Environment' (1996)

As described in Chapter 3, the long-term viability of the earth's biosystems can be seen as the ultimate determinant of human health in terms of sustaining life on the planet. A core concept in thinking about human-induced impacts on the natural environment has become sustainability. The term 'sustainable development' was coined in 1987 by the World Commission on the Environment and Development (Brundtland Commission) which concluded that economic development without attention to environmental constraints will, in the long term, threaten population health. Sustainability is premised on the principle that the rate of consumption of natural resources should be balanced with the rate that the earth is able to regenerate them (McMichael 2001). Time is a key factor in this equation. Communities that are sustainable are those living within their environmental means.[6] Those that do not are consuming resources at a pace that depletes the earth's capacity to sustain life. There are clear inequities, with high-income countries consuming a disproportionate share of the world's natural resources and contributing more than their fair share of pollution. The Netherlands, US, Japan and Israel are among the worst offenders as measured by the size of their ecological deficits (Wackernagel and Callejas 1995). The average American produces six tons of carbon dioxide, a Chinese person 0.7 tons and an Indian person 0.25 tons per year (Brown 2002c).

There is increasing evidence that current forms of globalization are accelerating the rate of environmental change. Since the Industrial Revolution, human activity has added 170 billion tons of carbon to the atmosphere, with a 2 per cent annual growth in emissions. Current concentrations of CO_2 are higher than at any time in the past 150,000 years (Flavin 1996). Meanwhile deforestation has continued apace, driven by the global trade in forest products rising from US$29 billion in 1961 to US$139 billion in 1998 (French 2000: 20). Similar pressures are being placed on the world's mineral, water and land resources. According to the Living Planet Index (LPI), natural wealth of the planet has declined 33 per cent between 1970 and 1999. This rate of decline, about 1 per cent annually, is unprecedented in human history. At the same time the ecological footprint, a measure of the changing human pressures on the natural environment over time, has increased by 50 per cent from 1970 to 1997, a rise of 1.5 per cent per year. This level already exceeds the biosphere's regeneration rate (WWF 2000). Similarly, according to surveys by the World Conservation Union (IUCN), an estimated one-quarter of the world's mammal species and 13 per cent of plant species are threatened with extinction (as cited in French 2000: 9).

Perhaps the best documented evidence comes from global climate change. Research has so far focused on gradual changes such as the natural waxing and waning of ice ages over millions of years or, more worryingly, human-induced warming of air and water temperatures over hundreds of years from the increased emission of greenhouse gases. However, there is emerging evidence that gradual changes have been punctuated by episodes of abrupt change including temperature changes of about 10° C (18° F) within a mere decade in some places. Severe droughts or floods have marked such abrupt changes, as well as accompanying impacts on human civilizations. For example, some glaciers in Alaska are now melting at an 'exceptionally high rate', with at least 8 per cent of the sea level rise in the past decade due to the thinning of their mass by several hundred feet. Climate warming is believed to be one of a number of factors controlling glacier mass balance, including local climate and glacier geometry (Arendt et al. 2002). Importantly, abrupt changes have been especially common when the climate system is 'forced to change most rapidly'. Hence, 'greenhouse warming and other human alterations of the earth system may increase the possibility of large, abrupt, and unwelcome regional or global climatic events' (US National Academy of Sciences 2001: 1). Current evidence suggests we may be in the midst of such a change, with six of the ten warmest years recorded occurring in the last ten years, the other four occurring in the 1980s.

As well as contributing to such alterations, globalization is expected to spread the resultant effects more widely:

> With growing globalization, adverse impacts – although likely to vary from region to region because exposure and sensitivity will vary – are likely to spill across national boundaries, through human and biotic migration, economic shocks, and political aftershocks ... the issues are global ... (US National Academy of Sciences 2001: 7).

This is evident in the increasing number of people affected by 'natural disasters' over the past three decades. According to the ICRCRCS report (2002), the number of disasters rose from 1110 to 2742 between the 1970s and 1990s. The number of people injured or made homeless by disasters rose from 740 million in the 1970s to more than two billion in the 1990s (including double counting of those repeatedly affected). The estimated economic losses (at current values) have grown from US$131 billion to US$629 billion during the same period. An estimated 25 million people are displaced by environmental causes, more than double the 12 million political refugees. It is anticipated that a sea level rise of 0.5 to one metre would similarly affect millions in low-income countries such as Bangladesh, Nigeria, Egypt and Guyana, and make uninhabitable at least five island nations including the Maldives, the Marshall Islands and Tuvalu.

This 'new paradigm of an abruptly changing climatic system' high-lights the need for a greater sense of urgency to achieve more sustainable forms of globalization. The impacts on human health, and indeed the survival of the human species, will not necessarily be gradual or reversible. Current forms of globalization are worsening this impact by encouraging the spread of unsustainable practices to other parts of the world. While contributions to this alarming situation vary by individual and country, the rate at which we are collectively impacting on the natural environment merits more timely action.

4.8 Conclusions

When scientists began to decode the human genome in 1995 they estimated it would take about ten years to complete. The publication of the final version in 2003, two years ahead of schedule, is not the result of progress in biology but advances in computer technology. The 3.12 billion 'letters' of the human genetic code were mapped by hundreds of computers at sixteen centres around the world. The exponential growth of computing power has been a major boon for medical research because it enables the automation of mundane and time-consuming tasks (e.g. data crunching). This has led to a new branch of science, bioinformatics that applies computer-assisted analysis to biological systems (Harvey 2000a).

These rapid advances by the Human Genome Project illustrate the opportunities to health from technologies that enable more rapid capacity to store, manipulate and reassemble large amounts of information. Health is one of the most information-intensive sectors, and can thus benefit dramatically from these advances. For example, accurate and comprehensive record-keeping is central to health care. Patient records need to be updated regularly with information from various practitioners, cross-referenced for potential contraindication, and comparable to allow analyses of trends in population health. In some countries, there is a shift towards the 'paperless practice' but in most, patient records are manually maintained (Harvey 2000b). Information technologies can speed this process and allow fuller information to be stored and manipulated about individuals and population groups.

Information technologies also have an important role in medical research. Computers are used increasingly to simulate human organs, such as the heart, to speed the testing of new drugs; 'the machine can accelerate trials enormously, both by 'fast-forwarding' the simulation of the drug's effects and by eliminating some of the need for human guinea-pigs' (Harvey 2000b:20). Drugs testing can be speeded by the internet which allows data to be collected more quickly from a wide range of sites on patient responses to treatments, and more frequently using automatic monitors (Harvey 2000b:20). Literature searches can be conducted far quicker through electronic databases such as Medline and Popline. Many hours and days spent locating journal articles on site in a medical library can now be done by logging on and doing database searches in minutes. In the UK, OMNI (Organizing Medical Networked Information) is an initiative to provide a gateway to 'evaluated, quality Internet resources in health and medicine, aimed at students, researchers, academics and practitioners in the health and medical sciences'. The dissemination of health research has been quickened by faster processing of manuscripts by publishers using new information technologies to communicate with authors and publish materials electronically.

Hence, along with the spectre that certain health problems, such as infectious disease, can manifest and spread more quickly, globalization may bring the tools necessary to respond to them in a more timely manner. Influenza is a perfect example of the age-old race against time between humans and viruses. The history of influenza, perhaps dating as far back as Hippocrates, tells us that it has long been a pandemic disease, able to spread across the world within a matter of days. It is known as the fastest changing virus. In most years, influenza remains a relatively mild illness caused by a minor change in the virus (antigenic drift). However, there is the periodic prospect of a major change (antigenic shift) in the virus that produces a far more virulent strain to which people have no immunity. This occurred with devastating effect in the so-called 'Spanish flu' pandemic in 1918–19 when an estimated 20–40 million people died (see Box 2.3).

The actual rate of spread of infection is affected by a number of factors, notably the virulence of the virus, and the balance between immune and susceptible populations. The 1977–78 influenza epidemic in the US, for example, spread at about one-tenth of the rate of the 1918–19 variant in spite of vast differences in modes of transport and hence human mobility (Pyle 1986: 2). Since 1947, continuous monitoring of the virus for antigenic shifts has been undertaken by a worldwide network of institutions coordinated by WHO. According to WHO's Global Management and Control of an Influenza Pandemic (WHO 1998a), an improved international response has focused on enhanced human and veterinary surveillance, improved, low-cost, laboratory surveillance techniques, increased laboratory safety capabilities, enhanced electronic communications about influenza, enhanced vaccine production capabilities and access to antiviral agents.

The rapid isolation and characterization of influenza strains, in particular, is necessary for the development and distribution of effective vaccines. Each year WHO distributes newly detected strains to vaccine manufacturers. Using standard methods of vaccine production (growth of the virus in fertilized chicken eggs), the pharmaceutical industry orders millions of fertilized eggs up to a year in advance to ensure sufficient supplies, and can produce and distribute a vaccine in about six months. When an especially virulent strain emerges unexpectedly, however, with the capacity to pose a serious risk to a wider age group (up to 50 per cent of the world's population), it can take many weeks to build up enough stocks of eggs to start producing a vaccine (Firn 2001). Hence, there is concern that public health authorities would not be able to obtain sufficient vaccine stocks in time, and there would likely be a worldwide shortage when the next serious pandemic occurs.

> [I]t may well be, as it was in 1918, that a new pandemic will start in the United States. Moreover, even if the disease first appears in other parts of the globe, there may not be sufficient time to prepare enough of the immunizing agent to protect a sufficiently large segment of the population.
>
> (Weinstein 1976:1060)

Most recently, this occurred during the Beijing 'Asian A' influenza outbreak of 1993 when vaccine supplies ran short. The development of a new method of producing influenza vaccine by the Belgian company Solvay, using dog kidney cells, could if approved by regulators enable manufacturers to start producing virus (used to make vaccines) as soon as they are isolated by scientists (Firn 2001).

According to historical data, an antigenic shift is overdue. This heightened sense of concern lay behind the swift handling of two separate outbreaks of avian influenza in Hong Kong in 1997 and 2001 that resulted in the slaughter of 1.4 million and 1.2 million birds respectively as a precautionary measure. It has long been believed that the main source of major mutations in the influenza virus is the domestic duck of southern China, which is a natural carrier of avian flu viruses. From birds, the virus is believed to be transmitted to domesticated pigs and then humans. The habitation at close quarters of bird, pig and human populations in the region facilitates this process. What remains unclear is how globalization may be changing the likelihood of a virulent strain of influenza emerging, and how quickly it might spread worldwide. A far greater understanding is needed of the potential links between the intensification of food production methods, increased trade in food products, and shifting demographic patterns in the region and beyond, and patterns of antigenic drift and shift in the influenza virus. Otherwise, as Leahy (2001) reports, 'whenever Hong Kong's chickens sneeze, the rest of the world will be at risk of catching the flu.'

Similar types of internet-based networks have been set up, or are sup-ported, for a range of surveillance, monitoring and reporting applica-tions. In 1994–5 the value of the Salm-Net surveillance system and its links outside of Europe was demonstrated when the rapid exchange of information enabled the identification of the source of a major out-break of *Salmonella agona* in Israel and associated cases in North America (Killalea et al. 1996). An EU-funded evaluation of the arrange-ments for managing epidemiological emergencies involving more than one EU member state concluded that existing networks to detect inter-national disease outbreaks are essential and need further expanding (Brand et al. 2000). The process of revising the International Health Regulations by WHO, whose importance was illustrated by the SARS (Sudden Acute Respiratory Syndrome) outbreak in 2003, also relies on such networks of government and nongovernmental organizations to provide timely and accurate information about outbreaks, information that has not always been available in the past.

In short, the temporal challenges posed to health by globalization push us to harness the very technologies driving change to respond to them. This is already happening most notably in the area of infectious disease control. Other applications – remote sensing of global environ-mental change, drugs testing, clinical reviews, telemedicine – are far ranging and rapidly developing. Given the scope of this book, these cannot be covered here. Nonetheless, the key element of time is clear in all of them. The importance of ensuring that there is a shared capac-ity to use these technologies is also clear. Effective responses to many global health issues, by definition, require all population groups to contribute to their resolution. A global network for infectious disease, for example, is weakened overall by an inability of poor countries to participate. It is this shared interest in strengthening health systems worldwide that is perhaps the most pressing challenge ahead.

Key Readings

Anderson R. and R. May (1991), *Infectious Diseases of Humans, Dynamics and Control* (Oxford: Oxford University Press).

Gleick J. (1999), *Faster, the Acceleration of Just About Everything* (New York: Little, Brown).

Levine R. (1997), *A Geography of Time* (New York: HarperCollins).

Schlosser E. (2002), *Fast Food Nation* (Harmondsworth: Penguin).

5
The Cognitive Dimension of Global Health

Humankind has finally bid farewell to that world which could with some credibility be seen as a cultural mosaic, of separate pieces with hard, well-defined edges. Because of the great increase in the traffic in culture, the large-scale transfer of meaning systems and symbolic forms, the world is increasingly becoming one not only in political and economic terms ... but in terms of its cultural construction as well; a global ecumene of persistent cultural interaction and exchange. This, however, is no egalitarian global village.

Ulf Hannerz, "Scenarios for peripheral cultures" (1991)

5.1 Introduction

While the spatial and temporal dimensions of globalization readily receive attention by scholars and policy makers, how globalization affects the way we think is equally relevant for understanding its consequent health impacts. Indeed, the old adage 'you are what you eat' could be prefaced with the phrase 'you are what you think' because so much of what we do, including our dietary habits, is shaped by our beliefs, values, cultural attitudes and other thought processes. What we think, and hence what we and others do to affect our health, is being continually shaped by the environment around us. As the nature of this environment becomes increasingly global, so too are the influences on our thought processes. It is this cognitive dimension of globalization that this chapter explores.

The study of human cognition is a well-established and multidisciplinary endeavour embracing such diverse fields as psychology, sociology, cultural and media studies, and neuroscience. It is beyond the scope of this chapter to pay sufficient due to the range of theories and empirical findings of this body of work. It is useful, however, to scope out in broad terms some of the ways that globalization is influencing human cognition:

- Since the 1980s the telecommunications sector has been deregulated and privatized across almost all countries. These policies have been spurred by a desire to encourage the growth of the sector, as the core infrastructure underpinning a post-industrial global economy, through competitive markets and private sector investment.
- There has been a greater concentration of ownership of communications by large private corporations that operate transnationally. Horizontal and vertical integration has increased in the hardware or infrastructure that enable the production and distribution of communications (that is, computers, service providers, telecommunications), and in the software and content of the messages produced and sent (that is, film, radio and television programmes, advertisements, popular music, literature, news, research).
- An increasingly global industry in the production of research and policy is emerging in the form of consultancy firms, think tanks, corporate research arms, academic and specialist publishers, educational institutions and international organizations that increasingly operate transnationally.
- Trade in cultural goods – printed matter, music, visual arts, cinema, photography, radio and television – has increased exponentially over the past three decades (UNESCO 2000). For some, this is seen as contributing positively to the emergence of a 'global village', increasingly united in shared cultural experiences, as well as enhanced democratic and participatory possibilities. For others, this is seen as a process of 'cultural imperialism' that extends the economic and political dominance of Western civilization (notably the US) to the rest of the world.
- Globalization has itself become a discourse within which competing schools of thought are struggling to influence the minds of policy elites and public opinion.
- More people worldwide have ready access to information and communication technologies (ICTs) than ever before, notably in the form of television, telephone and computer. Furthermore, much of this technology is linked to global networks through satellite and cable technologies. However, there are clear inequities in access to such technologies between the 'information rich' and 'information poor' within and across countries.

The products of human cognition, and the means of communicating them, are especially central to the health field. Historically, exclusive control of specialist knowledge, and its application under formal licence, has underpinned the legitimated power and status of the medical professions. Today, such knowledge runs through all facets of health policy and practice – as the basis of planning and priority setting within health systems, as core messages in health promotion, as inputs in the development of new interventions and treatments, as the means of ensuring informed consent by patients, and as the basis for understanding patterns of health and disease. The movement to support 'evidence-based practice' in recent years is a reinforcement of the central role of certain forms of knowledge in making health-related decisions. The increased popularity of systematic reviews, meta-analyses, treatment protocols, and information clearing-houses reflect this focus. Furthermore, health continues to be one of the largest sectors of research across most countries, prolifically churning out scientific and scholarly papers for thousands of specialist journals and publications each month. Public interest in health matters is also intense, as witnessed by the amount of coverage given to health stories in the mass media, and by the fact that health is the most popular type of information sought on the internet. The health field, in short, is driven by a wide range of cognitive processes.

This chapter focuses on five key areas of cognition that, as a result of globalization, are influencing human health. The first concerns the global influence of policy ideas surrounding health sector reform since the early 1980s. These ideas have clear origins in neoliberal principles that initially took hold in the US and UK, but gradually spread throughout the public sectors of many countries. Second, and relatedly, widespread efforts to improve priority setting in public health have been strongly informed by certain globalized discourses. To a large extent, neoliberalism has played a defining role in elevating decision making based on economic rationale. Since the late 1990s, the theme of global health security has also become increasingly popular, invigorated by the events of 11 September 2001. Third, the importance of epistemic communities surrounding scientific research is examined. The risks to the integrity of independent research is considered in light of how globalization is extending the reach of vested interests into the research community through changing patterns of funding and other activities. Fourth, the globalization of marketing and advertising is explored in terms of their impacts on behaviours and lifestyles that, in turn, have consequences for human health. Finally, the emerging consensus around global health ethics is discussed in relation to their effect on health research, public policy and corporate activities.

5.2 The globalization of health sector reform: from Health for All to pay your own way

We cannot adopt a system in which the macroeconomic and financial is considered apart from the structural, social and human aspects, and vice versa ... What is new is an attempt to view our efforts within a long-term holistic and strategic approach where all the component parts are brought together ...

James Wolfensohn, President of the World Bank (1999)

Poverty eradication is now the menu, but the main dish is still growth and market liberalization, with social safety nets added as a side dish, and social capital scattered over it as a relish. Big government is not available as an option ... the bank is rushing round the world eradicating poverty by signing up countries for programmes which have poverty in the headline but all the usual World Bank conditions about market liberalization in the small print.

The Nation (Bangkok), 5 July 2000

The health sector in countries around the world has been the target of intensive reform since the 1980s. Admittedly health sector reform is a more ongoing process than the term suggests, whereby governments in all countries periodically reflect on, and adjust, aspects of national health systems to meet changing needs. Nonetheless, a clear movement to substantively reform the health sector began in the US during the 1970s. The impetus for reform has nominally been a desire to find better ways of providing and financing health care, including the promotion of efficiency, equity and effectiveness (Frenk 1994). This has been spurred by emerging epidemiological and demographic trends and, not least, a shifting ideological climate. In the US, where total expenditure on health as a proportion of GDP is about 14 per cent, Republican administrations introduced various means into the largely private health care system to control costs, focused on reducing the role of hospitals, encouraging greater competition among insurers and providers, limiting the range of services covered, and increasing out of pocket payments (Marmor 1994). In the UK, successive Conservative administrations introduced their own vision of reform to the National

Health Service (NHS). Policies introduced during the 1980s and 1990s include an internal market, fundholding by general practitioners (GPs), autonomous hospital trusts, and tax incentives to encourage private insurance and service providers (Paton 1997). Other industrialized countries followed suit, notably New Zealand (Devlin et al. 2001) and Canada (Ruggie 1996).

Importantly, the health reforms pursued have been an extension of a set of policy ideas known loosely as neoliberal economics or, as Williamson (1990) coins, the 'Washington Consensus'.[1] While the pace and sequence of such reforms continue to be a subject of keen debate within the US government, multilateral development banks, IMF, think tanks and academia, the approach remains strongly committed to the creation of well-functioning markets as a precursor to economic development. The Washington Consensus formed the backdrop to the reform of health systems worldwide and, it is argued in this chapter, represents a form of cognitive globalization that is having profound impacts on health. The reforms introduced to public services as a whole over the past two decades have been aimed at delivering greater efficiency, responsiveness and flexibility. Its advocates argue that governments had grown too large and unwieldy, needing instead to pull back from the direct provision of many public services including health care. A minimalist role for government is envisioned that involves guiding and facilitating socioeconomic development, rather than actually implementing policy decisions (a 'hidden' rather than 'invisible' hand). The latter would be left to private sector actors within a competitive market. The ideas behind this paradigm shift became known as 'new public management' (NPM) or 'new public administration' (Kaul 1997).

It is beyond the scope of this section to review the broad range of health sector reforms tried and tested in countries around the world based on NPM ideas.[2] These are briefly summarized in Box 5.1. In the context of this chapter, what is of interest is the lineage of such ideas and how they have come to be disseminated globally via certain interests and processes. What explains this take-up of similar reforms across high, middle and low-income countries? Is it due to a convergence of health needs and challenges across the world? This is unlikely given the diversity of national and local contexts involved, and the continued difficulties of defining clearly their specific needs and priorities. Is it the sheer logic and practical effectiveness of NPM ideas in meeting these needs? This too seems unlikely given the limited evaluation of such reforms during the period of their speedy introduction, and the unavoidably uneven results found in analyses since the late 1990s (Schick 1998). Indeed, the global nature of health sector reform since the 1980s lies not so much in the convergence of practice around a proven and effective set of policy ideas, but rather the global forces defining the particular reforms undertaken and then driving their adoption in so many countries.

The transfer of similar packages of health reform to the developing world came within the wrapper of structural adjustment programmes (SAPs) introduced by the World Bank from the early 1980s. As a part of the conditionalities attached to Bank loans, governments throughout Asia, Africa, Latin America and, from the mid 1990s, central and

---

Box 5.1   New public management and health sector reform

Health care financing
- performance or output-oriented planning policies and procedures
- shift from cash-based accounts to accrual accounting
- charging of capital investment in assessing real cost of health services
- decentralization of budgets to purchasers
- increase in private health insurance
- introduction of co-payments (e.g. user fees)
- liberalization of health insurance market

Health care service provision
- reconceptualization of health service users as active consumers
- demands of consumers used as cues for health service to be more responsive
- delineation between health policy formulation and implementation functions
- separation of funders, purchasers and providers of health care
- establishment of minimum standards of health care and compilation of data on quality of care
- identification of basic or core health services package
- competition among service providers
- flexible staffing and recruitment practices
- introduction of incentives that encourage achievement
- performance agreements specifying outputs to be provided
- contracting out of health services (non-clinical and clinical)
- development of partnerships with private for-profit and private not-for-profit sectors

Source: Compiled from M. Kaul (1997), 'The New Public Administration: management innovations in government', *Public Administration and Development*, 17: 13–26.

eastern Europe, were required to adopt some or all of the following policy prescriptions:

- reduce public expenditure on health (and other social sectors);
- reduce the size of the health system by circumscribing available services and privatizing selected services;
- reduce the size and increase the efficiency of the workforce in the health system through retrenchment, downsizing and performance-related pay;
- introduce alternative and additional sources of financing such as user fees, private insurance and foreign investment;
- create quasi-markets through, for example, multiple health care providers, contracting out, commissioning, separation of purchasers and providers of health services, and fundholding; and
- restructure the health system to encourage more accountability such as decentralization and autonomous hospitals.

By the mid to late 1990s, accumulating evidence of the decidedly uneven results of neoliberal economics in the developing world, punctuated by severe financial crises in parts of Asia and Latin America, led to a reassessment of the appropriateness of such policy prescriptions. Most notably, it was recognized that policies aimed at creating functioning markets alone were one of the prerequisites, not an end in itself, in development. While such policies can contribute to economic growth in countries with relative equity, strong institutions, institutional capacity, and democratic governance, they can worsen conditions in countries without such preconditions (Weisbrot et al. 2001). As described by Joseph Stiglitz (1998), former Chief Economist of the World Bank and fierce critic of IMF policies following the Asian crisis: 'we have broadened the objectives of development to include other goals, such as sustainable development, egalitarian development, and democratic development. An important part of development today is seeking complementary strategies that advance these goals simultaneously.'

Widespread evidence that neoliberalism was having adverse effects on health, particularly the health of the poor within and across countries, led to similar reflection. For example, gains in health status by Zimbabwe during the 1980s were pointedly reversed by the introduction of the economic structural adjustment programme (ESAP) during the 1990s (Loewenson 2000). The introduction of user fees in countries such as Kenya, Papua New Guinea, Tanzania and Niger were shown to have led to drops in health-care use, raising concerns about knock-on public health risks (for example STDs, reproductive health). Rather than generating increased resources for health, so-called 'cost-sharing' was substituting and not supplementing public expenditure, resulting in an inadequate resource base to finance essential health services (Jowett 1999). Similarly, the introduction of user fees for water supplies in South Africa, as part of the country's SAP, led to a serious outbreak of cholera in 2000 (BBC News 2001). Under current negotiations of the General Agreement on Trade in Services (GATS), major trading powers such as the European Union are pushing for the liberalization of water utilities[3] along with other public services. This is raising further fears that, in a world where 1.3 billion lack access to clean water, and where inadequate access to sanitation contributes to 12 million child deaths annually, such a policy will have grave consequences (Watkins 2002)

Recognition of the importance of the social sectors to economic development has been an important lesson for the emerging 'post-Washington' Consensus. The relationship between better health and economic development was a core message put forth by Gro Harlem Brundtland then WHO Director General, after taking office in 1997. Seeking to elevate health on national and global policy agendas, she recast health from a 'non-productive' social cost to an essential investment for enabling effectively functioning economies amid globalization: 'health must be seen as a central factor not only in social development, but also in countries' ability to compete on the global economic stage and achieve sustainable economic progress' (Brundtland 2001b). To support this policy shift, a WHO Commission on Macroeconomics and Health (CME), chaired by former Harvard University Professor Jeffrey Sachs, was formed in 2000 to undertake studies on 'how concrete health interventions can lead to economic growth and reduce inequity in developing countries'. It was also mandated to recommend 'a set of measures designed to maximize the poverty reduction and economic development benefits of health sector investment' (WHO 2000d).

The language used in health policies worldwide has converged around this reframing. Since the mid 1980s, economists and public health experts within the World Bank have supported health policies informed more strongly by economic rationale. The seminal Global Burden of Disease Study (GBD) based at Harvard University (Murray and Lopez 1996) was the flagship analytical effort to underpin this new approach (Box 5.2). Criticism of its starting assumptions, methodological rigour and implicit political agenda elicited fierce debate between the public health community, largely focused around WHO, and health economists centred around Washington DC (Lee and Goodman 2002). Admittedly, the lines of ideological and analytical allegiance were far more complex. Yet it was clear that there was a clear difference in philosophical starting points between those who remained committed to health as a human right versus those who supported the use of economic rationalism to inform decisions about the distribution of health resources.

The change in paradigm since the late 1990s has favoured the latter. Among the new staff recruited by Brundtland when she resumed office were Christopher Murray and Alan Lopez, the former becoming Director of the Global Programme on Evidence for Health Policy in 1998 and Executive Director of the Evidence and Information for Policy Cluster in 2001. Professor Richard Feachem, former head of the health division at the World Bank and major contributor to the *World Development Report: Investing in Health* (World Bank 1993), became editor of the *Bulletin of the World Health Organization* in 2000. Critics joked that Harvard University and the World Bank now had a branch office in Geneva.

Whether or not criticism that WHO has been co-opted is justified, there has been an observable convergence in the arguments mustered by WHO, the World Bank and other health-related organizations around efforts to boost the profile of health on high-level policy agendas. The search for good investments, in terms of health gain per dollar spent, now preoccupy health economists worldwide. League tables ranking various burdens of disease by disability adjusted life years (DALYs) have been taken up by governments around the world as the basis for making allocative decisions. Calculations about the cost-effectiveness of different interventions for each is then being fed into the concept of a 'basic package' of health care that each country is encouraged to provide. All the time, the message that investing in health is prudent economics remains centre stage:

- Higher household incomes enable individuals and societies to achieve better health. But it is also true that better health contributes to higher incomes. Hence, health status is a significant predictor of subsequent economic growth (Bloom and Canning 2000).
- For every 1 per cent of HIV prevalence in a country that has an excess of 10 per cent, there will be 1.5 per cent annual decrease in GDP per capita. When countries have 8 per cent or more infected, the loss of national income is estimated at 0.8 per cent of GDP per annum (World Bank 2002).

Box 5.2   The Global Burden of Disease Project

The lack of accurate and comprehensive health data over time and across all populations around the world remains an enduring problem. Poor health information at the national and global level weakens decisions about, for example, priority setting and targeting of specific populations. The Global Burden of Disease (GBD) Project was a five-year effort, beginning in 1992 and funded by the World Bank, with the aim of compiling epidemiological information on a wide range of diseases, injuries and risk factors. Researchers at the Harvard School of Public Health and WHO, with more than 100 collaborators worldwide, produced estimates of patterns of mortality and disability for eight demographic regions, along with projections to 2020. As described by its authors, the ten-volume study offered 'the first comprehensive picture of the world's current and future health needs'.

An important feature of the project was its development of an approach to measuring health status that quantifies, not only the number of deaths, but also the impact of premature death and disability on a population known as disability adjusted life expectancy (DALE) and disability adjusted life years (DALYs). These were combined into a single unit of measurement known as the 'burden of disease' on the population. The project also provided the first estimates of the proportion of mortality and disability that can be attributed to certain risk factors for disease including tobacco, alcohol, poor water and sanitation, and unsafe sex. The study revealed a number of startling observations including the underestimation of the burden from mental illnesses, the deteriorating health status of men in the former Soviet bloc countries, and the expected role of tobacco by 2020 in killing more people than any single disease. The vast amounts of data generated by the project fed directly into the World Bank's *World Development Report: Investing in Health* (1993), seen by many as seminal in shaping thinking about international health priorities since the mid 1990s. Since the project, refinement and extension of the GBD data and methodology has been carried out in relation to individual countries and health conditions, and has informed the work of the WHO Commission on Macroeconomics and Health.

Despite claims of its being a 'comprehensive, internally consistent and comparable set of estimates', there have been ongoing and vigorous debates about its methodology. Critics have focused on three issues. First, it is argued that the quality of the data used in the project has been so weak as to undermine the results of the study. Second, the methodology is seen by many as deeply flawed in its economic assumptions in terms of moral and ethical values. The stronger weighting given to economically productive members of society and, by extension, lesser weighting given to children and older people, means different value is given to the health of these populations. Third, the practical relevance of the measures for poor countries has been questioned. While the methods claim to work towards the rational

---

Box 5.2   continued

identification of a basic health-care package for individual countries, combining the heaviest disease burden with the most cost-effective interventions, more fundamental issues about weak capacity and lack of resources are not addressed.

Source: C. Murray and A. Lopez eds (1996), *The Global Burden of Disease* (Cambridge, Mass.: Harvard School of Public Health/Oxford University Press); A. Williams (1999), 'Calculating the global burden of disease: time for a strategic reappraisal?' *Health Economics*, 8(1): 1–8.

- Africa's GDP would be US$100 billion greater if malaria had been eradicated 35 years ago. Malaria slows economic growth today by 1.3 per cent annually (Jha and Mills 2002).
- Tuberculosis causes a loss of US$12 billion per year from the incomes of poor communities (Brundtland 2001b).

In some respects, the political agendas of the left and right in health appear to have converged, notably around the needs of the poor. In recognition of the disproportionate burden that macroeconomic reforms can inflict on the poor and vulnerable, there is now an admission that greater attention is needed to providing debt relief, 'safety nets' and other pro-poor measures. Almost universally, the World Bank, health-related UN organizations, and bilateral aid agencies such as the UK Department for International Development (DfID), have realigned their aid budgets towards poverty reduction (Short 2001; World Bank 2001; SIDA 1997; Natsios 2001). Other shared goals include the need to create 'capable states' rather than merely reducing the size of states, including the achievement of an appropriate 'mix' of the public and private sectors.

However, despite greater consensus about the importance of health development including poverty reduction, there remain clear theoretical differences about how these should be achieved. The World Bank remains wedded to the promise of poverty reduction through economic growth achieved by trade liberalization, market forces, and global economic integration (Dollar and Kraay 2000). Critics see these as part of the problem, rather than the solution, and call for redistributive policies that ensure greater social justice and socioeconomic equity.[4] Furthermore, the division between those who deploy an economic rationale for health development, and others who support a human rights approach based on ethical and moral principles of universalism, remain evident. There is growing concern that a global health policy has emerged which is too steeped in the language of economic utilitarianism. For many, this is a betrayal of the principles of Health for All adopted by WHO in 1978 that all people are entitled to basic health rights, and society (government) has a responsibility to ensure such rights.

In summary, the principles of neoliberal economics that have redefined the role of the state and the market since the 1980s have been directly evident in health sector reforms undertaken by countries around the world. The global reach of NPM policies has been achieved through national governments, bilateral aid agencies and multilateral institutions searching for effective ways of addressing the changing health needs of both the industrialized and the developing world. Importantly, the uptake of these ideas was not only the result of coercion, although it is clear that policy conditionalities were imposed on many low- and middle-income countries. More fundamentally, NPM ideas have become globalized, in the sense that they have been legitimated in high-level policy circles within all of these institutions. While there remains fierce debate about the rights and wrongs of NPM, the parameters within which the search for a post-Washington Consensus is taking place are clearly delineated.

5.3   Priority setting in global health policy: whose agenda?

Failure to establish a process for priority setting or serious deficiencies in this process have led to a situation in which only 10% of research funds from both the public and private sectors are devoted to 90% of the world's health problems.

Global Forum for Health Research, *The 10/90 Report on Health Research* (2000)

If a virus or bacterium were killing as many people as tobacco does, that would be cause for general panic ... Our most basic challenge may therefore be cultural: we need to find ways to value our public health. Once we have done that, tolerating tobacco won't make any more sense than tolerating smallpox or polio.

Anne Platt McGinn, 'The Nicotine Cartel' (1997)

As described above, health has been at the heart of policy debates around public sector reform since the 1980s. As well as being a traditionally large recipient of public spending in many countries, thus competing with other sectors for scarce resources, the cost of health care has risen substantially over recent decades. Ageing populations, the availability of new and expensive medical interventions, the increased cost of drugs and, in some countries, the challenge of emerging and re-emerging infectious diseases (ERIDs) have all contributed to greater pressures on the public purse. Internationally, levels of official development assistance (ODA) have fallen since the 1990s, and the regular budget funds (RBFs) of WHO continues to be constrained by the practice of zero real growth exerted by major donor countries (Vaughan et al. 1995).

The need to set clear priorities is a core function of policy making. In health policy, to some extent, priorities can be set by the clinical decisions of individual practitioners about the most appropriate treatment for patients. A more strategic process, however, involves such activities as setting health targets, carrying out annual spending reviews, costing of interventions, and evaluating programmes in terms of whether they meet health needs. An idealized priority setting process might be one based on an objective analysis of the relative burden of various health conditions, the availability of different interventions, and the relative cost of health care.

In reality, there has been much criticism of the way in which health priorities have been, and continue to be, set by the international community. Historically, the needs of the Great Powers of the US and Europe circumscribed international health cooperation throughout the nineteenth century to focus on those countries' trade and geopolitical interests. Health sector aid after the Second World War was strongly shaped by the Cold War, as well as by links with formerly colonized territories. Even today, many bilateral aid agencies continue to favour certain parts of the world because of historical links rather than absolute need. The UK Department of International Development, for example, is committed to achieving the International Development Targets (IDTs) in the poorest countries of the world 'where there is a coincidence of high levels of poverty, poor health status and meager national resources' (UK DfID 2000). However, 13 of the top 20 countries receiving bilateral health aid from the UK are former British colonies, and some countries on the list, such as Pakistan, Brazil, Russian Federation and China are not among the poorest nations in the world. Similarly, USAID has traditionally favoured Latin America, and parts of Southeast Asia and the Middle East for strategic reasons rather than an objective assessment of health need. In the case of the

Japanese International Cooperation Agency (JICA), there has been a preference for providing high-level, often inappropriate and preferably nationally-produced technologies and hospital infrastructure, rather than recurrent costs.

Different UN organizations have had their own systems for setting health priorities, to a certain extent driven by competition for scarce resources as the UN system came under criticism from the mid 1970s for its effectiveness. The debates over comprehensive versus selective PHC reflected fundamental differences in priority setting approaches. The Health for All by the Year 2000 movement was launched in 1977 by WHO and UNICEF and was seen as a major breakthrough in public commitment to the human rights approach to good health. Its emphasis on providing comprehensive primary health care was lauded for its shift in focus away from expensive and often inappropriate interventions. However, within a short time, HFA was being criticized for giving inadequate direction to priority setting. UNICEF began to pursue a selective PHC approach under its GOBI-FFF[5] initiative that prioritized certain interventions notably oral rehydration therapy (ORT) and child immunization. While WHO continued to advocate the development of broadly based PHC systems, UNICEF successfully attracted substantial public funds to undertake its GOBI-FFF initiative under charismatic Executive Director James Grant. Grant's legacy was to create a clear and positive image in the public's mind about the work of the organization, and to focus on feasible and measurable (some would say relatively easier) interventions. For many, however, UNICEF was guilty of 'showboating' and doing only the relatively easy and photogenic tasks, like immunizing children, while leaving the harder and longer-term struggle of building health systems to other organizations. Similarly, UNFPA struggled to find its place in the UN pecking order especially given the controversy over its role in national family planning programmes. The high-profile International Conference on Population and Development (ICPD) held in Cairo in 1993 put forth the term 'reproductive health' as a framework for defining priorities in the population field. However one decade or so after the conference, many argue that the term has still not been transformed into sufficiently clear priorities for action.

The importance of catching the public's imagination has been an important influence on priority-setting for NGOs as well. Certain population groups, such as women and children, tend to evoke a more sympathetic response by the public than, for instance, elderly people, intravenous drug users or commercial sex workers. Also, the perception of an individual as a 'victim', because of their weak position in society, the occurrence of natural disasters or other circumstances beyond immediate control, is more powerful at mobilizing support for their health needs than if their situations are seen as self-inflicted (such as smokers). Other problems, such as the rapid spread of Hepatitis C since the late 1980s, mainly through the use of dirty syringes, has become a neglected global crisis because of its association with intravenous drug users (IDUs). Many NGOs have become skilled at resourcefully taking advantage of these emotional responses, even to the extent of 'marketing' selected human tragedies for public consumption. The penchant by the mass media for 'news' has complemented these tendencies, focusing disproportionate attention on humanitarian crises and emergencies, rather than the need for long-term investment in health systems.

> our media bosses expect us to meet a bottom line, a certain profit margin, a given stock market flow. And in order to do so we have to be catchy, be there twenty-four hours a day, be there all of the time. Total access! We are there in your living room. And what suffers in the atmosphere of immediacy is analysis. What suffers in this search for speed is depth. The media in the wealthy world are becoming increasingly simplistic, superficial, and celebrity-focused (Garrett 2000).

Not surprisingly, perhaps, private-for-profit companies set their business plans on the basis of expected financial return on their investment in various health interventions. In doing so, this has led to the problem of so-called 'orphan drugs' or 'neglected diseases'. Many medical interventions are not financially attractive for pharmaceutical companies to develop, perhaps because sufferers are primarily among the world's poor or because the condition occurs among a relatively small population group. These include malaria, kala-azar, sleeping sickness and tuberculosis, all diseases that afflict large numbers in the developing world but do not hold the promise of large financial returns.

The process of priority setting for global health, therefore, falls far short of being a rational and transparent process. There are clear anomalies. In a study of the role of extrabudgetary funds to WHO, Vaughan et al. (1995) found that aid donors strongly favoured programmes concerned with infectious diseases that have traditionally garnered greater public support over less attention-grabbing needs such as health systems development. The neglect of noncommunicable diseases (NCDs), despite accounting for an estimated 40 per cent of deaths in the developing world and 75 per cent in the developed world (19 million total deaths worldwide annually), is another example (WHO 1996a). At the same time, data by Gwatkin et al. (1999) remind us that focusing on the so-called epidemiological and demographic transition towards NCDs in industrialized countries neglects the needs of the world's poor. Infectious diseases continue to cause 60 per cent of death and disability among the poorest 20 per cent of the world's population. Similarly, the Council on Health Research for Development (COHRED) has drawn attention to the striking 10/90 gap[6] in how resources for health research are allocated worldwide.

In recognition of the need for better priority setting, there have been numerous efforts since the 1990s to improve the information base upon which such decisions are taken, encourage better coordination of efforts among key institutional actors, mobilize new resources, and create new institutional configurations. The first task, improved data for priority setting, has been led by the above discussed Global Burden of Disease Project which seeks to provide a more rational way of measuring and comparing different health needs. Drawing on these data, a Five-Step Process was proposed by the Ad Hoc Committee on Health Research beginning with GBD data to identify priorities. The Advisory Committee on Health Research argues for priority to be given to 'problems of critical significance to global health' and where the need for action is 'imperative'. In May 1998 the World Health Assembly adopted a resolution supporting a new strategy of Health for All in the 21st century which identifies ten 'global health targets' as the world's most important health issues. In identifying these targets, WHO seeks to create a shared vision and motivate member states to take action and set priorities for resources (WHO 1998b). Again, the use of GBD data lies at the heart of this process based on the principle that 'our recommendations should be based on evidence rather than ideology' (WHO Director-General Harlem Brundtland as quoted in WHO 2000d).

An alternative framework put forward for priority setting is the concept of global public goods (GPG) for health. In formal terms, a public good is one that is nonrival (it can be consumed without becoming depleted) and nonexcludable (no one can be barred from consuming it). A lighthouse, clean environment and national security are classic examples of public goods. GPGs are 'goods whose benefits reach across borders, generations, and population groups' (Kaul et al. 1999: xxi). It is argued that processes of global change have extended public 'goods' and 'bads' to the global level because of the extended reach of their externalities. In the health field, therefore, 'policy-makers must be concerned about health in jurisdictions other than their own and about policies that could encourage externality-producing countries to internalize their spillovers' (Kaul 2001: 79). However, public goods in general tend to be under-produced without collective action, due, for instance, to the free rider problem. The 'juris-dictional gap' between the global nature of some health issues and national focus of policy decisions and action is also a key challenge. The lens of GPG for health, therefore, seeks to identify priorities by explaining important gaps in global health cooperation, and identify what actions would provide the most collective benefit. These priority areas include infectious disease prevention, control and treatment; epidemiological monitoring and surveillance of infectious diseases; and health information.

The focus by the GPG approach on issues that create externalities beyond national borders is consistent with definitions of 'global health' that put the preoccupations of high-income countries at the forefront. In its 1997 report *America's Vital Interest in Global Health*, the Institute of Medicine states that the 'movement of 2 million people each day across national borders and the growth of international com-merce are inevitably associated with transfers of health risks, some obvious examples being infectious diseases, contaminated foodstuffs, terrorism and legal or banned toxic substances'. The report goes on to state that positive externalities, in the sense that 'healthier populations abroad would also constitute more vibrant markets for U.S. goods and services', were an important motivator. Laurie Garrett's *The Coming Plague* (1994) effectively drew wide attention to the risks posed to industrialized countries from emerging and re-emerging infectious dis-eases. Similarly, Kassalow (2001) writes that

> Emerging risks to the health and security of Americans make it prudent policy to grant higher priority to health in these countries. In addition to the threat of the deliberate spread of disease through biological weapons, Americans may now be at greater risk than at any time in recent history from recognized and emerging infectious diseases. These diseases are resurgent everywhere and spread easily across permeable national borders in a globalizing economy. The proliferation of drug-resistant organisms makes diseases more difficult to treat. The rising incidence of life-threatening chronic dis-eases in developing countries adds to the problem. Lack of attention

to the burden of disease in these countries, which receive 42 percent of U.S. exports, may depress demand for those goods and services and thus threaten the jobs of Americans.

This literature has been successful in ensuring that health is considered an important part of the post-Cold War agenda and a claimant to the so-called 'peace dividend'. As described in Chapter 1, health has become an agenda item in major forums such as the UN Security Council, G8 summit meetings and the World Economic Forum. More generally, health issues were found to rank first in Gallup's International Millennium Survey among concerns that matter most in people's lives (as cited in Kaul 2001).

Despite this welcome attention, concerns about how health issues have been framed within this emerging paradigm have begun to be expressed. In part, defining a clear agenda for 'global health' has been a genuine struggle over the meaning of terms such as 'global' and 'globalization' (see Chapter 6). However, it is also clear that there are inequalities in power over agenda-setting on global health, with dominant interests framed as globally shared. As Navarro (1999a: 221) writes,

> when WHO supports the recommendations of the Institute of Medicine's influential report, America's Vital Interest in Global Health, which calls for rich countries such as the United States to help in globalizing health policies, the question that must be raised is: *whose health policies?* Those of the commercial health insurance companies, or those of average families in the United States and other countries? They are in conflict.

The cost of focusing on those externalities that pose the greatest threat to the industrialized world is the distortion of priorities for political expediency. In terms of burden of disease, tobacco-related diseases, injuries and mental health are all major challenges for global health that dwarf morbidity and mortality from biological weapons. Other fundamental challenges, such as the development of effective health systems, do not even register on the radar of high-level policy makers because they do not fall into the category of a 'clear and present danger'.

The emerging agenda around public health security is a good example of national interests driving contemporary efforts to define global health priorities. The links between health and foreign policy are long established but limited in scope. The International Sanitary

Conferences held during the nineteenth century, for example, were ostensibly aimed at facilitating economic and trade relations between European powers and their colonial territories. Since the Second World War, health sector aid has been a major component of ODA provided by high-income countries to the developing world, undoubtedly to address health needs but also to further geopolitical goals. The rapidly emerging paradigm around public health security since the late 1990s, accelerated by the events of 11 September 2001, and bioterrorist spread of anthrax in the US, illustrates how global health can become a part of prevailing foreign policy. As Fidler (2002) writes, *Realpolitik* has taken strong hold of American foreign policy and, along with it, any vision of collective global health cooperation. With the protection of national self-interest as the foremost principle, the US government's primary target is combating terrorism, shoring up domestic preparedness, and engaging in international cooperation only where national interests are served. Consequently, perceptions of risk from the threat of biological and chemical weapons, for example, albeit a real one, have been given disproportionate attention relative to other health risks (RAND 2002).

The need for good governance to support priority setting will be critical in coming decades as new resources are being raised for global health initiatives. 'New' philanthropists such as the Bill and Melinda Gates Foundation, UN Foundation and Soros Foundations Network, accompanied by renewed government commitments, bring much needed resources to global health. The creation of the Global Fund to Fight HIV/AIDS, Tuberculosis and Malaria in 2001 (Box 5.3) follows numerous other public–private partnerships and initiatives aimed at targeting specific health needs (Buse and Walt 2000). Even before the fund was announced, the challenges of structuring its governance to decide priorities and allocate resources became immediately apparent. After the decision to prioritize malaria, tuberculosis and HIV/AIDS in the first instance, other decisions need to be made. What criteria will be used to assess proposals to receive support from the fund? How many resources will go to drug and vaccine development versus health systems? Which countries will be given priority and on what basis? For some, the fund represents a return to the disease-focused era of vertical programmes from the 1950s to 1970s. For others, it represents a new type of partnership of international organizations, governments, civil society and the private sector needed to tackle global health issues in the twenty-first century.

Box 5.3   Global Fund to Fight HIV/AIDS, Tuberculosis and Malaria

At the Group of Eight (G8) Summit held in Okinawa, Japan, in July 2000, and a follow-up meeting of health experts in December 2000, it was agreed that a fund be created to strengthen global efforts to fight HIV/AIDS, tuberculosis and malaria. Amid increasingly large anti-globalization protests at major international meetings, the G8 Summit held in Genoa in July 2001 confirmed the initiative as a means of demonstrating the commitment of world leaders to addressing the needs of the developing world. The three diseases kill an estimated six million people each year, primarily in low-income countries. An estimated US$10 billion per annum is needed to meet the goals of the Fund. As of mid 2002, US$2 billion had been pledged by governments, charitable foundations, private citizens and businesses. Major contributors include donor governments, Kofi Annan, the Bill and Melinda Gates Foundation, European Union and UN Foundation. Further contributions have been slow to appear, as donors wait to see how effectively the Fund achieves its goals.

There is much interest in how the Fund relates to existing national and regional programmes, to NGOs, and to global initiatives and international organizations such as the WHO and UNICEF. Careful attention was urged from the onset about who would be eligible for support and how proposals would be assessed. In October 2001, a 40-member Transitional Working Group (TWG) met for the first time, charged with the task of setting out the parameters of the Fund's structure and functions including its management structure, implementation process, accountability and financial systems. Its composition included representatives of low-income countries, donor governments, NGOs, the private sector and the UN system. Regional consultations followed shortly after in Asia, Africa, Eastern Europe and Latin America, along with meetings with NGOs and the academic community to solicit wide-ranging views on how the Fund should be run.

In late January 2002, an 18-member Board of Directors met for the first time, composed of 14 seats divided equally between low-income and donor governments, and two seats each for the NGO (one each from a low-income and high-income country) and private sector (one each from a private foundation and private company). The term on the Board is two years, with each constituency responsible for selecting its own representatives. WHO, UNAIDS, the World Bank and a person living with or affected by HIV/AIDS, TB or malaria have additional ex-officio non-voting seats. The Board is headed by Professor Richard Feachem, former Dean of the London School of Hygiene and Tropical Medicine and former head of the Health Division at the World Bank. A small secretariat based in Geneva manages the flow of work and supports the Board, while the World Bank acts as Trustee with primary responsibility for financial accountability. An independent 17-member technical review panel reviews and recommends proposals for support to the Board.

Overall the Fund is described as an independent public–private partnership for leveraging resources for countries and groups with the highest

---

Box 5.3 continued

disease burden and need for financial resources. The Fund supports pro-grammes for strengthening health systems and country-level partnerships involving governments, the private sector and civil society. In addition, the Fund supports the purchase of critical health products such as bednets, condoms, anti-retroviral drugs, anti-TB and anti-malarial drugs. A total of US$616 million over two years was awarded to 58 programmes in 43 countries in its first round of grants.

The creation of the Fund has been welcomed by the health community as a source of much needed resources for three major diseases. At the same time, concerns have been raised about the disease-focused nature of the Fund's work, recalling debates around vertical versus horizontal approaches to health development. The NGO community has also expressed worries that it is not clear how the Fund's activities will fit with national policies and poverty reduction strategies, as well as concerns about the sustainability of the initiative, the capacity of national health systems to absorb the resources, the risk of distorting national priorities and, perhaps most funda-mentally, whether priorities remain too donor-led.

Source: Compiled from Global Fund to Fight AIDS, Tuberculosis & Malaria website <www.globalfundatm.org> and Bretton Woods Project (2001), 'Global health fund debated' <www.brettonwoodsproject.org/topic/social/s23health-fund.html>.

In short, priority setting lies at the centre of current debates around the emerging policy agenda for global health. While there is a general reluctance to use the term 'rationing' in relation to health care, in reality all health systems must set priorities, given limited resources and virtually unlimited demand. The important question is how priorities are set, by what criteria, and for what costs and benefits. These are both technically and politically difficult ques-tions. Existing systems to govern this process have led to clear anomalies within and across countries. The recent penchant for evidence-based decisions has led to a competitive 'battle' of mortal-ity and morbidity statistics whereby the more people you can claim your health issue kills or disables, the greater priority you can try to obtain. There is some validity in such an approach. But of course, it has never been, and perhaps never will be, a question simply of how many people are affected. Normative factors – ethics, moral values, custom – invariably come into play, and a more transparent and equitable system to govern the weighing up of such considerations is essential.

5.4 The role of scientific research: the transnational power of epistemic communities

It's the responsibility of the university to serve the public good. The public relies on universities for the greatest degree of objectivity, rather than for information that may be slanted by financial interests.
Nils Hasselmo, President of the Association of American Universities (as quoted in Kowalczyk 2001)

*We would aim to place an article every two months in one or other of the WSJ [*Wall Street Journal*], the* Times, *the* Telegraph, *the* Spectator, *the* Financial Times, *the* Economist, *the* Independent *or the* New Statesman.
Professor Roger Scruton, email to Japan Tobacco International (as quoted in Maguire and Borger 2002)

In the specialized and highly technical field of health, the role of scientific research is critically important. Health research generates information and knowledge for policy and practice, as well as basic understanding of the determinants of health. The image of the white-coated scientist peering down a microscope in a laboratory for the good of humankind is an enduring one. However, health research today is a broad church, embracing the natural and applied sciences, as well as the social sciences, and humanities. The wide range of research feeding into contemporary health policy and practice stems from recognition of the broad determinants of health.

The elevated role of the expert has correspondingly developed alongside the importance given to health research. The health field, perhaps more than any other, is characterized by its strong epistemic community defined as 'a network of professionals with recognized expertise and competence in a particular domain and an authoritative claim to policy-relevant knowledge within that domain or issue-area' (Haas 1992: 2). The role of epistemic communities does not stop at the hallowed halls of academia but extends to policy-making circles. Given traditional deference towards the 'medical mafia' (Pitt 1992) and other health professionals, non-members of that epistemic community can find it difficult to challenge the views of health expertise. Indeed, since the late 1990s, there has been a strong movement to further strengthen 'evidence-based' medicine by more closely integrating clinical practice with the best available scientific evidence.

Implicit within this movement is a strong positivist perspective that assumes health research is value-neutral, cumulative and progressive. Positivism or rationalism posits that

> there exists a reality driven by immutable laws. Science seeks to discover the true nature of this reality, the ultimate aim being to discover, predict and control natural phenomena. Investigators are shaped by the belief that they are detached from the world ... Knowledge about the world is then summarized in the form of universal, or time- and context-free, generalizations or laws (Pretty 1994: 37).

The idealized image of health research is thus that it is independent of vested interests and carried out for the benefit of society as a whole. Academic institutions, for example, have an important role to play. As stated in UNESCO's Declaration on Higher Education (1998), higher education institutions should 'use their autonomy and high academic standards to contribute to the sustainable development of society and to the resolution of the issues facing the society of the future' (UNESCO 1998).

Critical analysis of health research is needed for a number of reasons. First, the closer links between the public and private sectors since the 1980s raise questions about the fundamental purpose of some research. Spurred by a decline in public spending on higher education, as well as a push for more 'applied' or 'policy relevant' research, institutions have been under pressure to attract more private research funding. In the US, where this is particularly pronounced, private funding of academic research has grown 8.1 per cent annually since 1980 to US$1.9 billion in 1997 (Press and Washburn 2000). In the UK, 12 per cent of research income (£242 million) for higher education institutions came from industry and commerce in 2001 (Copeland 2002). Moreover, there are indications that the emergence of an 'academic–industrial complex' has global implications given the sources of funding and their research outputs.

A detailed analysis of the long-established and varied links between academia and the private sector is beyond the scope of this book. However, there are a number of concerns within the health research community that warrant examination in terms of their relevance to understanding the cognitive reach of globalization. While accurate data are notoriously difficult to obtain, it is estimated that R&D represent 3.4 per cent of annual expenditure (US$56 billion) on health worldwide. About 50.4 per cent of this figure is from government sources, 44.3 per cent from the pharmaceutical industry, and 5.4 per cent from the private not-for-profit sector such as charitable foundations (Michaud and Murray 1996). Notable since the mid 1990s has been a substantial increase in private sources of funding for health-related research, much of which has been given for global health campaigns. It is estimated that one-fifth to one-half of total industry R&D in basic biomedical discovery (US$50–60 billion) occurred within US universities in 2000 compared with about US$25 billion in government spending. An additional US$8–10 billion came from private foundations (Moses and Martin 2001). In many cases, public–private partnerships have formed as a means of leveraging greater resources but also to tap into sources of knowledge and expertise (Buse and Walt 2000). The extent of privately funded research is illustrated by the decision in June 2002 by the editors of the *New England Journal of Medicine* to relax its longstanding rules on conflicts of interest so that it can publish review articles and editorials about new drugs by researchers with minor[7] financial ties to manufacturers. The decision was taken because of the lack of experts without such ties, and the editors were concerned that doctors might rely exclusively on pharmaceutical companies for information about new treatments (Drazen and Curfman 2002).

The assumption that health research and expertise is value-neutral at worst, and value positive at best, is increasingly challenged by the globalization of vested interests that can influence health research. A more sinister form of influence is the use of expert status to access and shape public policy making, sometimes without appropriate declarations of potential conflicts of interest. The setting of occupational exposure standards in the WHO and ILO, for example, has been strongly criticized as influenced by corporate consultants acting on behalf of major chemical companies such as Bayer and DuPont (Castleman and Lemen 1998). The asbestos industry, in particular, has played an important role in drafting and defining guidelines for the use of asbestos, chlorofluorocarbon refrigerants and other dangerous substances through corporate consultants serving on the International Programme on Chemical Safety in WHO and ILO expert groups during the 1990s. The industry has also used front groups (such as the Asbestos Institute) to sponsor training workshops and other events in the developing world where stronger restrictions have yet to be adopted. These findings are supported by Bartrip (1998: 42) who concludes that weak and late regulations of asbestos use in the UK, long after the hazards were understood, were because of '"cosy" negotiations between asbestos manufacturers and civil servants'.

Other industries have been accused of similar tactics. Berlan and Lewontin (1999) question the multiple roles of scientists representing biotechnology companies:

> The genetic-industrial complex is trying to transform political questions into technical and scientific ones so that responsibility for them can be shifted on to bodies it can control. Its experts, dressed in the candid probity and the white coat of impartiality and objectivity, use the camera to distract people's attention. Then they put on their three-piece suits to negotiate behind the scenes the patent they have just applied for, or sit on the committees that will inform public opinion and regulate their own activities. It is a serious thing when democracy no longer has any independent experts ...

Lang (1998) questions the representation of the food industry on the Codex Alimentarius Commission (CAC), the intergovernmental body created by WHO and the Food and Agriculture Organization (FAO) in 1962 to ensure that internationally agreed food standards, guidelines, and recommendations are consistent with health protection. Similar criticism has been levied at the International Agency for Research on Cancer (IARC) for possible corporate influence and conflicts of interest in its reviews of saccharin, methyl tertiary-butylether and 1,3-butadiene (Castleman 1999).

The tobacco industry is perhaps the best example of the wide range of ways that private companies may seek to influence the scientific process. The adverse health effects of tobacco use have been clearly demonstrated by scientific research since the 1950s (Doll and Hill 1950). Nonetheless, in the early twenty-first century, tobacco use continues to rise exponentially, with tobacco the leading cause of premature death, killing more people annually than either HIV/AIDS, tuberculosis or malaria (see Chapter 3). Of critical importance for understanding this apparent anomaly is the tobacco industry's role in influencing what is publicly accepted as scientifically proven, how valid the evidence is seen to be, what credibility individual researchers and institutions are given, how the tobacco and health issue is framed, and what policy responses are accepted as legitimate to pursue. The extent of the industry's involvement in purposively shaping the above has come to light through internal industry documents released since the 1990s to the public as a result of US litigation. These documents reveal that the industry has been engaged, since the earliest scientific evidence on the harmful effects of smoking began to appear, in countering, mitigating, distorting and undermining the findings of such research.

For example, one tactic used by the industry is to reframe the issue in order to distract from the public health impacts (Box 5.4). Beginning in the 1950s, when claims were even made that tobacco was good for one's physical and mental health, the industry put forth varied messages to win the hearts and minds of the public. Importantly, these efforts have been global in reach. While initially focused on high-income countries, where the major markets for tobacco remained until the 1990s, the industry increasingly turned its attentions to undermining arguments of the public health risks worldwide as these markets declined. One key target has been WHO and its associated institution IARC which the industry sought to undermine with criticisms of its governance and science (Bero and Glantz 2000). The exposure of British Professor Roger Scruton for soliciting further payment from the industry in return for writing articles in prominent newspapers, such as the *Wall Street Times* and *Daily Telegraph*, explained his penning of a pamphlet for the Institute of Economic Affairs attacking WHO's Tobacco Free Initiative. Scruton also offered to divert attention from the health risks from smoking by comparisons with 'fast-food of the McDonald's variety, which seems to be addictive, is aimed at the young, is a serious risk to health, with a worse effect on life-expectancy than cigarettes, and, unlike cigarettes, has a seriously corrosive effect on social relations and family life' (Scruton as quoted in Maguire and Borger 2002).

The highly publicised exposé of individuals pales in comparison with the highly organized manner in which the tobacco industry has mobilized its influence of health research worldwide. Strategies deployed include the funding of academic posts, funding of research projects casting doubt on the harmful health effects of smoking, sending of representatives to scientific conferences to present industry-funded research, sponsoring of conferences on related topics, publication of industry-funded research in prominent medical journals, recruitment of prominent or established scientists to undertake similar activities, and the establishment of front organizations that cast doubt on public health research. Examples of the above are provided in Box 5.5.

As well as facilitating efforts to influence the scientific process, globalization has extended the reach of the recent backlash against health experts. Revelations such as the above have contributed to an increased questioning of health experts in terms of the reliability of their proscribed scientific knowledge and the vested interests that may

---

Box 5.4   The industry's framing of the tobacco and health issue since the 1950s

1950s–1970s
- smoking is not harmful to health and nicotine is not addictive
- smoking can be beneficial for reducing stress, increasing concentration and soothing sore throats
- smoking gives you social status and confidence

1980s
- smoking is a personal choice and the right of an individual
- smoking by women demonstrates their independence and gender equality
- advertising is only used to influence the choice of brands by existing smokers rather than to encourage new smokers
- the tobacco industry makes a substantial economic contribution to society

1990s
- smokers contribute a disproportionate share of funding for public services through high taxes
- second-hand smoke is not a health risk but a problem of indoor air quality and 'sick-building syndrome' requiring better ventilation
- smoking low tar and 'light' cigarettes is less harmful to health
- raising taxes on cigarettes harms poor people and encourages smuggling
- smoking is a symbol of economic development and modernity
- WHO, and its associated institutions such as IARC, are flawed organizations

Since the late 1990s
- tobacco control is a Western-driven priority imposed on the developing world
- anti-smoking policies will harm poor farmers in the developing world
- there is a genetic predisposition to tobacco-related diseases
- the health risk from smoking is trivial (e.g. like crossing the street) compared with other lifestyle choices (e.g. fastfood)
- the industry admits its past mistakes and has changed, including working against marketing to children
- regulators need to work with the 'legitimate' and 'socially responsible' tobacco industry rather than attacking it

---

taint their judgement. In Europe, strong public feeling in the wake of BSE and vCJD has stalled the extension of GMOs to other parts of the world. The globally organized protests by environmental, consumer and health groups demonstrate the vulnerability that can come from being a global player such as Monsanto. After a key meeting of European environment ministers in June 1999, where a moratorium on GMOs was agreed, knock-on effects were felt worldwide as Japanese brewers, Mexican tortilla manufacturers, US agro-industrial giants

Box 5.5   Selected examples of tobacco industry efforts to influence health research

Operation Berkshire – In July 1977 senior executives of seven of the world's largest TTCs met at Shockerwick House near Bath, UK, to discuss cooperation on a wide range of matters to counter growing efforts to link smoking and ill-health. Dubbing the highly secret plan as 'Operation Berkshire', the companies agreed a wide range of activities including joint industry research into the benefits of smoking, support for national associations of cigarette manufacturers, and the creation of an International Tobacco Information Centre (INFOTAB). These collective efforts were aimed at fostering a 'smoking and health controversy' that was known to be spurious but was aimed at clouding the scientific evidence against smoking.

International Agency for Research on Cancer (IARC) – The tobacco industry carried out a multi-million dollar campaign to undermine a large-scale epidemiological study on the relationship between environmental tobacco smoke (ETS) and lung cancer. The study was conducted by the International Agency for Research on Cancer (IARC), an agency established under the auspices of WHO.

International Life Sciences Institute (ILSI) – The institute describes itself as an independent NGO that 'advances the understanding of scientific issues relating to nutrition, food safety, toxicology, risk assessment and the environment by bringing together scientists, government, industry and the public sector'. ILSI is partly funded by the food and drinks industry. In 2001 WHO cited tobacco industry documents released in 1998, following a legal settlement in Minnesota, that showed tobacco companies providing financial support to ILSI for 'services rendered'. WHO accused the industry of using ILSI to undermine its tobacco control efforts by becoming involved in 'seemingly' unbiased scientific groups and thus 'manipulating the political and scientific debate concerning tobacco and health'. ILSI vigorously denied the allegations, arguing that what the tobacco industry intended did not prove it was actually achieved.

Source: Francey N. and Chapman S. (2000), '"Operation Berkshire": the international tobacco companies' conspiracy,' *BMJ*, 321, 5 August: 371-74; WHO (2001b), *The Tobacco Industry and Scientific Groups, ILSI: A Case Study* <www.who.int/geneva-hearings/inquiry.html>.

Cargill and Archer Daniels Midland, all demanded a separation of GM from non-GM crops. The value of Monsanto stocks quickly dropped from US$62 to US$38 within a few months.

More pervasively, McKinlay and Marceau (2002) argue that there has been an undermining of key aspects of physician authority as a result of the internet. To a large extent, doctors have gained their status from exclusivity over medical knowledge. The internet goes some way in breaking this exclusivity by providing access to large amounts of health knowledge. This questioning of health expertise has been evident in the decline in uptake of the MMR (mumps, measles and rubella) vaccine in the UK, for example (Lawrence 2001:11).

The role of scientific research in health remains a core one in terms of providing the necessary knowledge to underpin policy and practice. Independent academic research is also vital to the upholding of a fundamental freedom, namely the ability to express views and raise questions that may challenge the status quo. This freedom lies at the heart of intellectual integrity. However, the 'golden age of doctoring' and health research of the mid twentieth century (McKinlay and Marceau 2002) has been replaced by a greater questioning of funding sources, potential conflicts in interest, and ultimately the messages of health experts. In large part, this has been brought about by processes of globalization that extend the reach of epistemic communities and the consequences of their actions. This suggests the need for a renegotiation of the relationship between the scientific research community and the public.

5.5   The globalization of lifestyles: the health consequences of marketing and advertising

If you could just sell one bottle of Coca-Cola to every Chinese every day, you'd be rich.
Sir Richard Sykes, Chairman of GlaxoSmithKline, on the approach of the soft drinks industry to the market potential in Asia (as quoted in Pilling 1999a)

The international market opportunity is what will keep us a growth company for many years to come.
Geoffrey Bible, CEO Phillip Morris (as quoted in Somasundaram 1996)

The whole rationale of the advertising industry is to try to alter people's thinking and, in turn, their behaviour. Most often, advertising[8] is used to urge us to consume particular goods or services. But it can also be used more subtly to educate, inspire, empower, and persuade through the shaping of beliefs, values and attitudes. Both the public and private sectors rely heavily on advertising to get their messages across. This may be achieved through in-house activities, such as a public relations office, or through professional advertising agencies that specialize in creating and executing targeted campaigns.

Closely aligned with the emergence of a global economy, advertising agencies have become increasingly transnational in their activities and operations. In 1990 US$300 billion was spent worldwide on advertising (Wallack and Montgomery 1992). During the recession of the early 1990s, many companies shifted their sights to the creation of new markets in Latin America, the Middle East and Eastern Europe. Coca-Cola, for instance, increased its spending on advertising in Argentina by 34 per cent in 1994 (Todd Pruzan, MARS, 1994 as quoted in *Consumers International* 1997). What is notable about trends in advertising is not simply the sheer growth in volume and its concentration in certain industries, but the use of new communication technologies that allow advertisers to send their messages to global audiences. As Wallack and Montgomery (1992: 205) write, 'The result is an increasing trend toward "global" marketing and advertising. In contrast to international marketing, which makes an attempt to reflect differing customs and values in the countries, global marketing creates the same messages for all countries.' The creation of 'global brands' is one important strategy in supporting the emerging global market. In February 2001, Coca-Cola Inc. decided to use McCann-Erickson to handle its creative advertising globally rather than local advertising agencies, a reflection of the global emphasis of its operations. The result of this expenditure is 'the emergence of a global mass culture ... a single world-wide civilization' (Madison 1998).

This trend towards the globalization of advertising has profound implications for health. The most heavily advertised products internationally are processed foods, soft drinks, cigarettes, alcohol, pharma-

Table 5.1   World's top ten advertising agencies in 2000

Agency	Gross income (US$)
Dentsu	US$2.4 billion
McCann-Erickson	US$1.8 billion
BBDO	US$1.5 billion
Walter Thompson	US$1.5 billion
Euro RSC	US$1.4 billion
Grey Worldwide	US$1.4 billion
Worldwide	US$1.2 billion
Ogilvy & Mather	US$1.1 billion
Publicis	US$1.0 billion
Leo	US$1.0 billion

Source: Adbrands Company Profiles. <www.mind-advertising.com>

ceuticals and toiletries, accounting for 80–90 per cent of all international advertising expenditure in the 1980s (Wallack and Montgomery 1992). Unilever, with food brands such as Bird's Eye and Liptons, spent US$5 billion on advertising in 1993. The fast food industry spends about US$4 billion on advertising annually (Schlosser 2002). As described in Chapter 4, the health consequences of this rapid increase in the consumption of fast food in high-income countries are increasingly well documented.

One of the core tactics in advertising campaigns is to create aspirational desires by playing on the human desire for self-esteem and social status. This strategy has long been used by TNCs seeking to expand their markets by using images of affluent, modern and western lifestyles. However, such campaigns can have adverse health

Table 5.2   Top 20 global marketers expenditure, US$ millions (1998 and 1999)

Advertiser	Rank 1998	Rank 1999	Headquarters	Countries marketed to	Worldwide media expenditure US$ millions 1998	Worldwide media expenditure US$ millions 1999
*Unilever	2	1	Holland/UK	66	3646	3698
Procter & Gamble	1	2	US	68	4880	4693
*Nestlé	3	3	Switzerland	67	1851	1909
*Coca-Cola	4	4	US	69	1435	1533
Ford	7	5	US	51	2288	2422
General Motors	8	6	US	43	3263	4108
L'Oréal	5	7	France	47	1525	1570
Volkswagen	6	8	Germany	33	1353	1381
Toyota	9	9	Japan	44	1706	1725
PSA Peugeot Citroën	10	10	France	37	909	906
Sony	12	11	Japan	53	1394	1477
*Mars	11	12	US	37	1148	1139
Renault	14	13	France	31	765	809
*Philip Morris	13	14	US	49	2044	2125
Henkel	15	15	Germany	35	742	747
Nissan	16	16	Japan	39	1154	1184
*McDonald's	18	17	US	54	1230	1282
Fiat	17	18	Italy	26	666	651
*Danone Group	23	19	France	24	579	691
*Ferrero	21	20	Italy	34	608	630

*Company with direct health-related impacts.
Source: Compiled from *Adage Global*, 2 April 2002. <www.adageglobal.com>

consequences. The methods to market breastmilk substitutes by food manufacturers, such as the use of sales representatives dressed as health visitors, depiction of products as superior, and provision of free samples to new mothers and health professionals, elicited strong criticism during the 1970s. Many mothers decided to use baby formula over breastfeeding, often without appropriate access to hygienic means of preparing it. Other parents, unable to afford the recommended amount of milk powder, fed diluted formula to their babies leading to severe malnutrition and even infant deaths. Despite the adoption of the non-binding International Code on the Marketing of Breastmilk Substitutes by WHO and UNICEF in 1981, NGOs allege that compliance with the code by major companies such as Nestlé, Milupa and Mead-Johnson remains questionable. In its report *Breaking the Rules 2001*, the International Baby Food Action Network (IBFAN) cited proof of infractions worldwide by 16 baby food companies and several manufacturers of bottles and teats (IBFAN 2001).

Similar aspirational messages lie behind the widespread use of skin lightening products throughout Africa. Dating from the colonization of the continent by Europeans, but accelerated by increasingly global messages of particular standards of beauty, it has remained socially desirable to dress, behave and look like Europeans. Today, creams are sold in tubes like toothpaste, accompanied by advertisements claiming, for example, that 'Successful people use AMBI, the best skin lightening creams in the world, Fastest action AMBI' (Chisholm 2002). It has become common for advertisements outside beauty salons to depict light-skinned men and women with long straight hair. The products bleach and, if used extensively, weaken the structure of the skin. In other parts of the world, notably in multi-ethnic societies, the same desire lies behind the increase in demand by non-white women for cosmetic surgery. This increased demand is focused on a desire to alter physical appearance to look more Caucasian. Hence, rhinoplasty is popular to reduce, narrow or alter the bridge of the nose. Oriental women request operations to provide the 'double eyelid' or western eyefold. Black women seek liposuction to alter body shape. In a study of eyelid surgery among Asian American women, Kaw (as quoted in Branigan 2001: 10) writes,

As women, they are constantly bombarded with the notion that beauty should be their primary goal. As racial minorities, they are made to feel inadequate by an Anglo American-dominated cultural milieu that has historically both excluded them and distorted images of them in such a way that they themselves have come to associate those features stereotypically identified with their race (ie, small, slanted eyes, and a flat nose) with negative personality and mental characteristics.

Aspirational messages are also behind the astounding growth of the fast food industry. In the US during the 1950s, when the industry emerged, it offered many people the opportunity to eat in a restaurant for the first time. As Love (1995) writes, 'Working-class families could finally afford to feed their kids restaurant food.' The industry also plays on the desire of parents to make their children happy, linking up with other global companies such as Walt Disney, because parents 'want the kids to love them ... It makes them feel like a good parent ... only McDonald's makes it easy to get a bit of Disney magic' (as quoted in Schlosser 2002). With skilled marketing, accompanied by changing social structures (notably the rise in numbers of working mothers) and lifestyles, fast food restaurants conquered the US over the next three decades. McDonald's spends more on advertising than any other brand. Ninety-eight per cent of American schoolchildren recognize the character Ronald McDonald, and the 'golden arches' have become more recognizable than the Christian cross. The growth of McDonald's Restaurants is seemingly unstoppable, currently numbering around 25,000 in 100 countries. As part of its 'global realization', McDonald's opens an average of five new restaurants per day, with 85 per cent outside of the US. It now ranks as the most widely recognized brand in the world (Schlosser 2002).

The regulation of how harmful commodities are marketed worldwide is a further challenge posed by globalization. The tobacco industry is a good example of the effort devoted to influencing public opinion through advertising, marketing and sponsorship activities.[9] The massive investment in advertising worldwide has paid off for Phillip Morris. The Marlboro Man was voted the number one advertising icon of the twentieth century by *Advertising Age* (Yach and Bettcher 1999). In 1997 Phillip Morris made more profits from foreign sales than domestic sales for the first time (Hammond 1998). By 2025 the developing world is expected to provide 85 per cent of the world's 1.64 billion smokers, an increase of 72 per cent. Alongside efforts to influence research and policy (see above), TTCs have skilfully appealed to aspirations, notably among prospective young smokers, for social

Box 5.6   India's cola wars

'Rival soft drinks marketers Coca-Cola Co. and Pepsi-Cola Inc. are pitched for a summer battle in India. A battery of new ads, distribution deals and products will be unleashed on the Indian public over the coming months as the two attempt to imprint their dominance over copycat brands and each other.'

'The newest brand entrant is international lemon cola drink Pepsi Twist, which is likely to be branded Pepsi Aha ... In an effort to challenge Coca-Cola's Indian brand Thums Up, Pepsi will be injecting more global work – such as that starring popstar Britney Spears and footballer David Beckham – into its local ad showings. Its "Sumo" spot is already proving a hit with urban India.'

'Coke's CEO Alex von Behr unveiled details at a press conference this week of 50,000 "new outlets all over the country where our consumers can buy our entire range," plus another 3, 500 outlets in villages to drive growth in rural India, an area which feeds only 30% of the company's revenues. At the same time, it is changing the ad strategy behind Maaza, positioning the local fruit-based beverage brand as a health drink, "fortified with calcium". The new strapline, "Yaari dosti, Taaza Maaza" ("friendship and Maaza") targets mothers with a focus on strengthening the friendship between mother and child.'

'Looking further than the summer battle, Coca-Cola India is also making deep inroads in the ready-to-drink tea and coffee market particularly as, according to the company's findings, almost 80% of the Indian population favour tea and coffee drinks during the day. With an eye on the winter season which starts in November, the soft drinks giant is planning to launch the Georgia coffee brand, currently on sale in Japan. The company has already tested its vending machines in New Delhi, to decide on the final composition, positioning and pricing of the products.'

Source: Excerpts from Gupte S. and Gupta R. (2002), 'India's summer cola wars', *Adage Global*, 28 March. <www.adageglobal.com>

status while downplaying the harmful health effects. The sponsorship of sporting and cultural events is intended to create goodwill and product identification with exciting activities.

By sponsoring Formula One, respondents claimed it made them believe that Benson and Hedges was a big, major league, very power-ful brand with plenty of money. It also lent associations to the brand with young, fast, racy, adult, exciting, aspirational but attain-able environments.

(As quoted in Hastings and MacFadyen 2000)

As restrictions on advertising and marketing have come into force in a growing number of countries, TTCs have sought to circumvent them by innovative means. The use of logos on clothing and other products that potential smokers may use is increasingly widespread. The distribution of free samples and promotional materials, notably where young people gather, is widespread in the developing world (MacAskill 1999). The use of 'product placement' in major films creates the association between smoking and glamour,[10] a message that is globalized through the worldwide dominance of the American film industry. Overall, public image remains a core concern of an industry widely criticized in recent years for its unethical behaviour. Phillip Morris remains second to last in surveys of corporate reputation, despite a US$250 million advertising campaign including changing its name to Altria.

While the overt and covert activities of the tobacco industry are being increasingly recognized, those of the alcohol industry receive far less attention. In 1983 the World Health Assembly (WHA) recognized problems related to alcohol consumption as among the world's major public health concerns. Economic globalization has contributed to these problems in three ways: (a) trade liberalization has led to the dismantling of a variety of market arrangements that serve to restrain and structure alcohol consumption; (b) multilateral trade agreements and growth of global marketing media has reduced the ability of national governments to control local alcohol markets; and (c) alcohol production, distribution and marketing are becoming increasingly globalized with expansion particularly into low-income countries and countries in transition (Jernigan et al. 2000). Like tobacco, alcohol suffers from being seen as a 'non-issue' by many people, and efforts to curb alcohol consumption have been met with similar accusations of the 'nanny state' and infringement of individual rights.

In summary, marketing and advertising has been a key force behind the emergence of a global economy, shaping our demand for the goods and services on offer by creating social and cultural aspirations for certain lifestyles and behaviours. The global nature of these messages is clear. The advertising industry is highly professional and sophisticated, and is itself an increasingly global operation. The health impacts are wide-ranging. There are potential benefits from harnessing marketing techniques for health promotion (Box 5.7). However, the balance of resources is clearly on the side of large corporations that do not have the protection and promotion of health foremost in their minds. In

Box 5.7   An example of using global advertising for health promotion

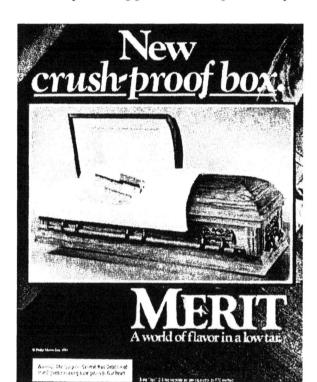

Source: Image reprinted with permission from Bonnie Vierthaler of The BADvertising Institute. <www.badvertising.org>

the present battle over the thoughts and actions of the public, there seems an inexorable trend towards globalized patterns of production and consumption.

5.6   Towards consensus on global health ethics?

Pfizer believes that globalization of clinical trials is key to establishing a worldwide standard of excellence in clinical trials and expanding access of novel medicines to patients around the world

(Pfizer 2000).

It's a new slavery, it's an economic slavery so that we in the West, we're all complicit in this, every one of us ... we're always looking for the cheaper product and it makes every company look for ways of cutting costs and the fastest way is to use child labour or sweatshop labour so we're all complicit.

Anita Roddick, Founder of the Body Shop (2001)

A wide range of ethical issues lies at the heart of globalization. Eschewing the view that globalization is somehow a natural process, the ethical challenges arising from its unfolding derive from the human choices that underpin its goals and the means selected to achieve them. An ethic, in simple terms, is a moral principle or set of moral values held by an individual or group. Collectively, ethics can provide a code of behaviour for a particular group, profession or individual to follow. Current forms of globalization, as defined in Chapter 1, are driven by certain values that, in turn, inform particular ideological assumptions and beliefs. In order to fully understand the nature of globalization, we need to make such values transparent and to consider their ethical basis in relation to their impacts on health.

The need for greater attention to ethical issues is strongly suggested by some of the features of contemporary globalization, many of which are described in this book. These include:

- inequalities of access to life chances and opportunities;
- an unequal shouldering of the costs of globalization by certain population groups, notably the poor and disadvantaged;
- a concentration of the benefits from globalization in a relatively small proportion of the world's population;
- evidence of unethical practices by some transnational actors;
- weak regulatory capacity to ensure good practice on a global scale;
- inequalities in political and economic power among global players;
- direct and indirect discrimination against certain populations on the basis of race, gender, disability and other unacceptable criteria; and
- lack of accountability and transparency within global public and private organizations.

In relation to the health sector, ethical issues arise from this global context in at least three main areas. The first concerns health research. Benatar (2001: 336) defines the challenge of research ethics in a globalizing world as 'how to construct universally valid guidelines for collaborative international medical research with the view to enhancing sensitivity to issues of justice and our common humanity'. In 1964 the Declaration of Helsinki was adopted to set out international standards for conducting medical research with human subjects. In 2000, the declaration underwent its fifth revision. Its provisions are clearly stated (Box 5.8) and, for the most part, research conducted in high-income countries are compliant with such principles, backed by nationally adopted codes of practice.

Box 5.8   Excerpt from the Declaration of Helsinki (1964)

1. Biomedical research involving human subjects must conform to generally accepted scientific principles and should be based on adequately performed laboratory and animal experimentation and on a thorough knowledge of the scientific literature.
2. The design and performance of each experimental procedure involving human subjects should be clearly formulated in an experimental protocol which should be transmitted for consideration, comment and guidance to a specially appointed committee independent of the investigator and the sponsor provided that this independent committee is in conformity with the laws and regulations of the country in which the research experiment is performed.
3. Biomedical research involving human subjects should be conducted only by scientifically qualified persons and under the supervision of a clinically competent medical person. The responsibility for the human subject must always rest with a medically qualified person and never rest on the subject of the research, even though the subject has given his or her consent.
4. Biomedical research involving human subjects cannot legitimately be carried out unless the importance of the objective is in proportion to the inherent risk to the subject.
5. Every biomedical research project involving human subjects should be preceded by careful assessment of predictable risks in comparison with foreseeable benefits to the subject or to others. Concern for the interests of the subject must always prevail over the interests of science and society.
6. The right of the research subject to safeguard his or her integrity must always be respected. Every precaution should be taken to respect the privacy of the subject and to minimize the impact of the study on the subject's physical and mental integrity and on the personality of the subject.

Source: World Medical Association (1964), *Declaration of Helsinki*. <www.ohsr.od.nih.gov/helsinki.php3>

However, in much of the developing world, where an increasing amount of health research is carried out, adherence to internationally recognized ethical principles is variable. Indeed, there is evidence to suggest that globalization is encouraging or at least enabling unethical practices. The cost of research in the developing world is much cheaper, and companies seeking to find savings in order to be globally competitive, may shift some of their research operations to Africa, Asia and Latin America. Relocating research also saves on costly delays in developing drugs,[11] and enables companies to get their products to the market much faster. The US Food and Drug Administration (FDA) has accepted new drug applications supported by foreign research since 1980. By 1999 27 per cent of applications contained a foreign test result, three times as many as in 1995. In South America, the number of researchers registered with the FDA to conduct experiments on drugs aimed at the US market increased from five to 453 between 1991 and 1999. Registered researchers in Eastern Europe increased during the same period from one to 429, and southern Africa from two to 266 (Flaherty et al. 2000). However, the capacity to monitor such research for compliance with ethical standards is weaker in many middle- and low-income countries. With financial pressures to test drugs more quickly and bring them to market, the pharmaceutical industry has discovered that the 'developing world is virgin territory, with millions of potential subjects' (Borger 2001).

The result has been alarming cases of bad practice. During the late 1990s, the German-based company Hoechst Marion Roussel (now part of the French-based Aventis Pharma) paid doctors in Argentina US$2700 per patient recruited for a trial of the heart drug cariporide. It was later discovered that for 80 per cent of the 137 patients recruited there were forged consent forms, and that 13 people had died during the trials between 1997 and 1998. While there is no evidence that the pharmaceutical company was involved in the deception, the case demonstrates the dangers of rapid expansion of clinical trials in the developing world. Similar public outcry followed revelations in late 2000 about Pfizer's clinical trials on children of a new antibiotic Trovan during a meningitis outbreak. The records of one 10-year-old girl, who died while receiving treatment with the unapproved drug while alternative treatments were at hand, drew particular chastisement. As reported in the *Washington Post*,

> Experiments involving risky drugs proceed with little independent oversight. Impoverished, poorly educated patients are sometimes tested without understanding that they are guinea pigs. And pledges

of quality medical care sometimes prove fatally hollow ... Drugmakers hop borders with scant government review. Largely uninspected by the [US] Food and Drug Administration – which has limited authority and few resources to police experiments overseas – U.S.-based drug companies are paying doctors to test thousands of human subjects in the Third World and Eastern Europe. (Stephens 2000)

In an effort to prevent such abuses, a report by the Nuffield Council on Bioethics (2002) identifies certain minimum requirements that must be met regarding research related to health care in low-income countries regarding informed consent, standards of care, activities after research is completed, and an effective system of reviewing ethical propriety. The vulnerability of certain population groups, such as children and the mentally ill, raises particular concern. However, the extent of poverty in the developing world means there is the potential for commercial exploitation of such populations on a widespread scale. More difficult is the question of whether it is ethical to use people for drug testing for a condition that is not prevalent among that population group. The testing of drugs for certain strains of HIV, for example, in Africa (where two-thirds of HIV-infected people live) that are prevalent in North America, Europe and parts of Asia has been criticized (Torassa 2000). Similarly, the ethics of developing treatments using people beyond whose financial reach the end product would be if it came to market, raises difficult moral questions. The strengthening of capacity in such countries to oversee compliance with international standards of medical research ethics is a key challenge (Singer and Benatar 2001).

As well as how health research is carried out, ethics are integral to the application of new scientific developments. Indeed, a number of new developments in medical research threaten to race ahead of thinking about their ethical implications. One example is recent advances in cloning. Cloning techniques range from the artificial splitting of embryos to produce genetically identical twins, to 'somatic cell nuclear transfer' to produce a genetic replica of a living organism (identical twin of a different age). The successful cloning of an adult sheep by Scottish scientists in 1997, in the form of Dolly the clone, triggered a raft of ethical debate about the application of the technique to human beings (Bettcher and Yach 1998). There are direct applications for health – cloning could be used to produce new tissue and organs with less risk of rejection. There is also a potential to apply the technology to fertility treatment (Trounson 1997). So far, efforts to extend this research to the cloning of human tissue have been resoundingly rejected on ethical grounds in the US and Europe. In other locations, where medical ethics is differently regulated, such research could proceed and then be shared worldwide.

The rapidly emerging field of genetics also brings with it a range of ethical challenges for the global community. The Human Genome Project provides a detailed map of the genetic makeup of human beings. This is expected to lead to revolutionary developments in the diagnosis and treatment of genetic disorders (see Box 4.2, p. 127). As more detailed knowledge about the genetic makeup of individuals becomes available, potential use by employers, insurance companies and other institutions raises concern that people will be unfairly treated. The prospect that one's life will become wholly predetermined by genetics, as depicted in the 1997 science fiction film *Gattaca*, is profoundly unsettling. How this knowledge is managed within a global information and communication system, therefore, has fundamental ethical considerations.

The rapidly advancing field of fertility treatment (also known as assisted reproductive technology or assisted procreation) is another minefield for global health ethics. The development of new methods, involving artificial insemination, *in vitro* fertilization (IVF), surrogacy, gene therapy and cloning, has steadily pushed the boundaries of procreation. In the US, the lack of federal government funding for such technologies has led to a highly commercial industry, worth US$2 billion annually, that falls outside laws that protect human subjects in research (Weiss 1998). Similar services are available commercially in Europe, Asia and elsewhere. The result has been a series of controversial cases that throw up unprecedented ethical and legal conundrums:

- In 2001 a 62-year-old French woman gave birth to twins following artificial insemination with a donated egg and sperm from her brother. The woman had not disclosed her correct age or the source of the sperm (Winston 2001).
- In April 1995 a baby was born in the US to a surrogate mother using an anonymously donated egg and sperm. The infertile couple, who had contracted the surrogate mother, sued for divorce one month before the baby was born, with the husband claiming no fatherly obligations. As the wife was neither the biological nor birth mother of the baby, and the surrogate relinquished her maternal rights by contract, the baby was born without legal parents (Weiss 1998).

- In Italy, considered by some as the 'wild west of assisted procreation', Dr Severino Antinori used IVF in 1994 to assist a 63-year-old to become the world's oldest woman known to give birth. He plans to develop methods of human cloning for fertility treatment, thus creating children with the same physical characteristics as one of its parents. Because of legislation banning human cloning in the US, UK and elsewhere, Dr Antinori is carrying out his research in an undisclosed location and on international waters. His colleague, American infertility researcher Dr Panos Zavos, predicted that a cloned human being would be born in 2003 somewhere 'between Greece and India' (D. Brown 2002).
- In April 2000 doctors in Saudi Arabia performed the world's first human uterus transplant from a 46-year-old woman to a 26-year-old woman. Reproductive organs are seen as the 'last frontier' of organ transplantation (Keith and Del Priore 2002).
- In March 2002, the UK Human Fertilization and Embryology Authority (HFEA) granted permission for an IVF clinic to use pre-implantation genetic diagnosis (PGD) to select an embryo free from disease and a genetic match for an existing sibling. The three-year-old brother of the planned baby, who suffers from a rare genetic blood disorder known as beta thalassaemia major, is expected to receive a bone marrow transplant using cells donated from the new baby (Horsey 2002).

In all of the above cases, technology has moved faster than societies' ability to address ethical considerations. Moreover, it is a commercial business that is increasingly transnational in its operations, because of the weakness of national regulations, giving rise to fears of 'procreative tourism'. Checks on the validity of information given by patients, the safety of procedures, and monitoring of compliance with prevailing ethical and moral standards all become more difficult to manage across borders.

Ethical decisions also underpin the making of global health policy in terms of allocative decisions about the types of activities to support and not support. As discussed in Section 5.3, priority setting in global health is a critical task for determining where resources and efforts are focused. Invariably, such decisions are strongly shaped by the value systems and beliefs of certain actors, such as aid donors. This, in turn, raises ethical issues regarding the ability of 'the piper to call the tune', thus extending value systems from one cultural context universally. The area of reproductive health illustrates this well. Since the early

1970s, there have been numerous clashes about the desirability and appropriateness of certain practices in family planning and population policies and programmes. To a large extent, this clash has been one of different value systems concerning the rights of women, the rights of the unborn, and the balance of these with the threat of unsustainable population growth. In 1984 these competing values came into direct conflict at the International Conference on Population held in Mexico City where the US government, supported by the Vatican, announced its withdrawal of funding to the UN Population Fund (UNFPA) on the grounds that it supported the provision of abortion services. A similar stance was taken by the Vatican at the International Conference on Population and Development (ICPD) in 1994 but the political climate had shifted in the US by this time under the Clinton Administration towards support for the concept of reproductive health. By the late 1990s, the pendulum had swung again, and efforts to expand the range of reproductive health services again met with opposition from the Catholic Church. For example, at follow-up meetings to the ICPD and Fourth World Conference on Women in 2000, the Vatican objected to the provision of the 'emergency contraceptive' (also known as the 'morning after pill') as a pretext for medically induced early abortion, as well as sexual relations outside of marriage (Tauran 2000). In May 2002, the US remained one of only two countries (along with Somalia) that has not ratified the UN Convention on the Rights of the Child (agreed in 1990) because its use of the term 'reproductive and mental health services for under 18s' could be seen to condone abortion. The Bush administration preferred the phrase 'reproductive health care' (Archibald 2002). In the context of the rapidly spreading HIV/AIDS pandemic in many parts of the world, the risks from other STDs, and the real dangers of unsafe abortions, the ability of one government to assert its value system in other countries through its relative wealth raises difficult ethical dilemmas.

Differences in main constituencies among departments within a single government can lead to contradictory, and some would argue unethical, policies being pursued at the global level. In terms of health ethics, the tobacco industry ranks among the most dubious. Its knowing production of a product that kills half of its consumers, its manipulation of the nicotine level of cigarettes to optimize addictiveness, its covert funding of front organizations (e.g. International Tobacco Manufacturers Association) to lobby on its behalf, its targeting of children and youth, its bribery of key officials, and its strategic undermining of public health researchers and institutions have all demonstrated the extent to which the industry will engage in unethical practices. Yet, while all of this has now been widely acknowledged in the public health community, many departments of trade and industry within the selfsame governments have protected and promoted the foreign markets of the tobacco industry. As well as sitting uncomfortably against domestic policies to reduce smoking rates, promoting cigarette exports can be juxtaposed with measures to stem the flow of illicit drugs into the US:

> *The U.S. exports huge quantities of tobacco to Colombia, Mexico, and other countries with whom it is continually wrestling to reduce the cocaine trade. Yet 40 times as many U.S. citizens die from tobacco use as from the use of all illegal drugs combined.*
>
> Ann Platt McGinn, *The Nicotine Cartel* (1997)

While the unethical behaviour of the tobacco industry is increasingly well documented, the activities of other global actors are also being examined. Globalization has enabled TNCs to extend their operations worldwide, sometimes to countries where public scrutiny is not possible and even discouraged. Indeed, companies may be attracted by more lax regulation of health and safety standards, working conditions and environmental protection, providing them with a competitive edge in the global economy. Many argue that this is resulting in a 'race to the bottom' whereby low-income countries compete for foreign investment by offering tax incentives, weaker social and environmental standards, and reduced protection and benefits for workers. The result, it is argued, has been the creation of 'sweatshop' conditions for many workers in the developing world, including the use of child labour, meagre wages and unsafe workplaces (ICFTU 1998). The ethical issues raised by these practices are clear. Major global companies, such as Nike, Disney and Gap have been accused of exploiting the world's poor by offering working conditions considered illegal in high-income conditions (Bruno and Karliner 2000). It is estimated by the ILO (2002) that 246 million children worldwide engage in forms of labour that should be abolished, including 170 million in hazardous work (such as mining, construction, quarrying) and 8.4 million in work likely to lead to irreversible physical and psychological damage (e.g. armed conflict, pornography). In China, for example, 'baby-face workers' earn about £2.25 for a 16-hour shift (Gittings 2001). Companies counter these accusations by arguing that such conditions are actually an improvement from prevailing standards in such countries, and that they offer work where otherwise there would be none. Many children work to support poor families, and the well-meaning introduction of workers rights comparable to high-income countries can lead to the loss of this important source of income.

While globalization is enhancing the ability of global companies to extend their operations worldwide, the capacity to scrutinize them more readily is also being facilitated. The ability to gather and share information, agree codes of conduct, monitor activities, mobilize campaigns and generate public awareness are all enhanced by the technologies of globalization. Campaigns led by civil society groups are, of course, nothing new. The worldwide boycott of the Swiss company Nestlé during the late 1970s and 1980s was the result of cooperation by NGOs based across many countries, coming together to form umbrella groups such as the IBFAN. Similarly, the movement to promote essential drugs lists in developing countries was strongly supported by a diverse range of civil society organizations. What is different today is the ability of such groups to network with like-minded groups, organize around a particular issue, mobilize resources and plan actions much more quickly and across a larger number of countries than ever before. A good example is the campaign against the proposed Multilateral Agreement on Investment (MAI). Negotiations centred on the 29 members of the OECD and remained a highly restricted process until the draft document was leaked by the Canadian delegation to the Council of Canadians, an NGO that opposed the agreement. The draft was quickly passed to Public Citizen and then circulated to other organizations worldwide. A mass campaign was soon under way which successfully led to the cancellation of the negotiations. As Mark Weisbrot, research director of the Preamble Center describes, 'This is the democratization of foreign economic policy. With the Internet, it's all more rapid. Before, the whole treaty wouldn't have been known about until it was too late to stop it' (as quoted in Longworth 1999).

This enhanced ability by civil society organizations to mobilize transnationally has led to greater pressure on big business and government to improve their governance. There is growing global consensus around certain standards of 'good practice', embodied in numerous codes of conduct and initiatives that organizations are encouraged to support (Box 5.9). Consumers International, the international federation of consumer associations, for example, put forth a Consumer Charter for Global Business in 1997 based on eight consumer rights: the right to basic needs, safety, information, choice, a fair hearing, redress, consumer education and a healthy environment. The Charter also sets out best business practice in ethical standards, competition, product standards, marketing, labelling, disclosure of information and consumer redress. It argues that good corporate governance goes far beyond corporate boardrooms and shareholder meetings, to include communities both domestically and abroad affected by their activities (Consumers International 2001). Corporate social responsibility (CSR) has become a keen subject of debate. Global campaigns to 'name and shame' companies, such as Disney, Nike, Nestlé and McDonald's, have been effective at generating bad publicity for image-conscious companies (Schwartz and Gibb 1999; Klein 2000). UN Secretary-General Kofi Annan has supported CSR through his call for a Global Compact, appealing to the business community to honour their social responsibilities, and harness the power of markets to make globalization a positive force for all (UN Global Compact Office 2001).

For the most part, health-related efforts to strengthen good practice amid globalization have been subsumed within this broader movement. As stated in the preamble to the Statement from Consumer International's 16th World Congress in South Africa in 2000, 'consumer rights and protection can only be achieved as part of a global struggle for justice for all people'. Similarly, health issues have been brought together with a wider agenda of social and environmental issues, strengthened by the number of organizations campaigning on their behalf and the collective voice they muster in the name of social justice. At the same time, however, there is a danger that health may become lost in what some see as an overly eclectic agenda, bound together by its opposition to the status quo but unclear in its vision of the desired change.

Nonetheless, the global agenda for health ethics is a growing one. The diversity of value systems and cultural contexts makes consensus on universal norms and values a major challenge. Yet there are clear minimum standards that are beginning to be recognized and slowly accepted, raising the level on what is seen as acceptable behaviour in health research, policy and practice. How well these efforts are translated into real change will depend much on the capacity to implement them especially in the developing world.

5.7 Conclusions

The adage that good health is as much about one's state of mind as one's physical condition takes on added meaning in the context of globalization. The cognitive dimension of globalization concerns

---

Box 5.9   Selected initiatives concerned with global health ethics

International Code on the Marketing of Breastmilk Substitutes (1981)
Following an international campaign and boycott against the company Nestlé, the Swiss company that employed unethical means to promote the use of baby formula, a code to regulate such practices was jointly adopted in 1981 by WHO and UNICEF. The Code has curbed but not eliminated inappropriate practices, and some companies are still found to be in breach of its stipulations. However, the issue has mobilized many civil society organizations, such as the International Baby Food Action Network (IBFAN), raised public awareness and served as a model for similar campaigns.

Social Accountability 8000
The first standard of social responsibility to be made fully operational by the NGO Social Accountability International <www.sa-intl.org> founded in 1997 as the Council on Economic Priorities Accreditation Agency (CEPAA). The standard is a workplace standard that covers all key labour rights and certifies compliance through independent, accredited auditors.

UN Consolidated List
Lobbying by Consumers International led to the creation in the early 1980s of the WHO Consolidated List of Products Whose Consumption and/or Sale Have Been Banned, Withdrawn, Severely Restricted or Not Approved by Governments. The list has been used by consumer groups to force governments to remove hazardous products from store shelves, and in some countries has led to the creation of systems for regulating hazardous products where none had previously existed.

Universal Declaration on the Human Genome (1997)
A declaration by the International Bioethics Committee of UNESCO as the first universal instrument in the field of biology. The agreement commits States to take appropriate measures to promote a set of principles that safeguard respect for human rights and fundamental freedoms, and the need to ensure freedom of research.

UN Global Compact (July 2000)
UN Secretary-General announces the UN's Global Compact containing nine principles dealing with human rights, labour and the environment whereby corporations are invited to declare their support for them. See <www.unglobal-compact.org>

World Business Council on Sustainable Development (WBCSD) see <www.wbcsd.ch>
The WBCSD is a coalition of 160 international companies with a shared commitment to sustainable development via the three pillars of economic growth, ecological balance and social progress. Members are drawn from more than 30 countries and 20 major industrial sectors. Its mission is to provide business leadership as a catalyst for change toward sustainable development, and to promote the role of eco-efficiency, innovation and corporate social responsibility. The organization states that: 'sound ethics and

Box 5.9   continued

core values offer clear business benefits accruing from the adoption of a broader world view enabling business to monitor shifts in social expectations and helps control risks and identify market opportunities. Such a strategy also helps to align corporate and societal values, thus improving reputation and maintaining public support.'

changes to the diverse thought processes that shape our daily lives. Where our thoughts come from, and the factors that influence them, have long puzzled scientists in a wide range of fields. Globalization brings an added complexity by introducing factors that flow across, and to a growing extent, disregard territorial boundaries. We are what we think, and what we think is increasingly global.

The capacity for globalization to open up new horizons in intellectual endeavour, scientific research and cultural creativity is full of promise for improving the quality of life of the human species. Health is a sector especially dependent on knowledge and information, and globalization brings opportunities to expand our understanding of health and health care, as well as to share this more readily with each other. Yet, we need to recognize that all cognitive processes are normative in their origin, and value-based in their application. This need not undermine their application to protect and promote health. Indeed, moral and ethical decisions should lie at the heart of health care. What is missing, however, is critical reflection of what is currently accepted as 'received wisdom' or 'common sense' about the priorities of global health and how they should be tackled. Many of the voices in current debates about globalization and health tend to hide behind the evidence base, claiming scientific objectivity or economic rationalism. Others preach from a moral high ground that fails to acknowledge the different realities of people's lives. How this impasse is resolved will hinge on changing how we think about global health which will invariably be a precursor to more effective action.

Key Readings

Collin J. (2002), 'Think global, smoke local: Transnational tobacco companies and cognitive globalization', in K. Lee ed., *Health Impacts of Globalization, Towards Global Governance* (Basingstoke: Palgrave Macmillan): 61–85.

Jackson J. (1998), 'Cognition and the Global Malaria Eradication Programme', *Parassitologia*, 40: 193–216.

Lee K. and H. Goodman (2002), 'Global policy networks: The propagation of health care financing reform since the 1980s', in K. Lee, K. Buse and S. Fustukian eds, *Health Policy in a Globalising World* (Cambridge: Cambridge University Press):

MacKay H. (2000), 'The globalization of culture?' in D. Held, ed. *A globalizing world? Culture, economics, politics* (London: Routledge and Open University Press): 47–84.

Bettcher D. and D. Yach (1998), 'The Globalization of Public Health Ethics?' *Millennium*, 27(3): 1–28.

6
Conclusion: An Agenda for Global Health

6.1 Introduction

This book attempts to provide a wide-ranging *tour de force* for understanding the impacts of globalization on human health. The conceptual framework developed in Chapter 1, and applied in Chapters 3–5, is intended to structure more clearly what is oftentimes a rather fluid and ill-defined subject. It is around this framework that copious examples have been provided to illustrate the diversity and complexity of this emerging subject area. This is an introductory text to encourage interest in, and provoke debate about, an emerging field of research, policy and practice.

Despite the varied content of the previous chapters, a number of crosscutting themes can be distilled from them that help to define an agenda for taking forward the challenges posed. This chapter takes us through these themes with the purpose of focusing some next steps that will help us better understand the changes occurring around us, and to strengthen the practical responses to them.

6.2 The importance of definition: from international to global health

> *What's in a name? That which we call a rose*
> *By any other name would smell as sweet.*
> William Shakespeare, *Romeo and Juliet* (1591)

> *You've got to name it before you can claim it.*
> Phil McGraw, *Life Strategies* (2001)

The frequent agonizing that academics engage in over definition and terminology is admittedly off-putting for those more inclined to concrete action. Seemingly esoteric debates, often within the confines of specialized disciplinary boundaries, about whether to use this term or that can seem mind-numbingly irrelevant to those who have the difficult responsibility of making decisions that affect people's lives. Whether one calls a phenomenon 'globalization' or something else understandably matters less than pursuing actions that harm the least, and bring the greatest good, to the most people. Hence, detailed discussion of the distinction between *international* and *global* health has a danger of succumbing to pedantic word games while the world succumbs to deadly pandemics, irreversible environmental degradation and deteriorating health systems. Surely the priority is to do something about what is happening rather than committing further intellectual energy to naming and renaming what we already know. Or is it?

One of the major hurdles for policy makers and practitioners seeking to take more decisive action on many of the issues described in this book is that of definition. If one of the first lessons in combat is to know one's enemy, the public health community is a muddled force for action. While some remain sceptical that globalization is anything new, others convinced of its newness cannot rigorously define what new quality it has. A varied collection of definitions has been offered, giving further ammunition to sceptics, or leading to people speaking at cross purposes. It then becomes impossible to know what we need to do to effectively manage what is happening. What actions do we need to take to promote and protect health? How do we know when we have successfully achieved this? What do we want and not want to change? What different state of affairs are we trying to achieve?

The starting point for this book has been that something distinct is happening in terms of health determinants and outcomes as a consequence of globalization. Globalization is historically located, as described in Chapter 2, but its contemporary phase is also particular to societies in the late twentieth and early twenty-first century. As a reminder, the definition used in this book is that globalization is a set of processes that is changing the nature of human interaction by the crossing of certain boundaries that have hitherto separated individuals and population groups from each other. These three types of boundary (spatial, temporal and cognitive) have become redefined, resulting in new forms of social organization and interaction across them.

A clear definition, in turn, is needed for the term *global health*, a term often used interchangeably with international health, or, more typically, to uncritically replace it. Without a clear definition, confusion arises as to whether the two terms represent fashion or a substantive shift in subject matter. What is *global* about global health? How is *global* health distinct from *international* health?

We can begin by clarifying the concept of health. The conventional definition of health focuses on the prevalence or absence of disease. However, the adoption of a broader and more positive notion of health by WHO upon its creation in 1948, as 'a state of complete physical, mental and social well-being and not merely the absence of disease or infirmity' (WHO, 1946), brought a new emphasis to well-being and social interaction. During the past half century, concepts of health have sought to define this more positive approach more precisely. Tarlov (1996:72) summarizes this thinking in terms of three conceptual components:

(a) health as a capacity to perform or function appropriately;
(b) health as a capacity to perform in order to achieve individual fulfilment such as the pursuit of tasks, values, needs and aspirations; and
(c) health as providing the potential to effectively negotiate the demands of the social environment.

Tarlov neatly summarizes these features into a definition of health as 'the capacity, relative to potential and aspirations, for living fully in the social environment'.

As well as defining what health is, a distinct concept of global health requires an understanding of the determinants of health. Put simply, the determinants of health are the full range of individual and collective factors and conditions, and their interactions, which correlate with health status (Health Canada 2000). Four broad categories are commonly identified as health determinants: (a) genes and biology; (b) medical care; (c) health-related behavioural risk factors; and (d) social characteristics (Tarlov 1996: 72–5). Recognizing that the last – social characteristics – is by far the most important, other schemata have been tried to separate out these more fully. Health Canada (2000), for example, cites 12 factors as determinants of health (Box 6.1)

If the determinants of health are seen as *cause*, and health outcomes or status as *effect*, global health can be understood as those impacts that globalization is having on both sides of this cause–effect equation.

Box 6.1   The broad determinants of health

income and social status – The economic resources available to an individual, and the status within a given society that an individual holds, directly influence level of health. On average, poor people are less healthy than rich people because of inability to afford enough nutritious food, quality health care, education and other basic needs. The greater the gap between the richest and poorest people within a society, and between countries, the greater the differences in health.

social·support networks – The strength of support an individual receives from families, friends and communities is linked to better health. Social support enables individuals to deal with difficult situations and contributes to positive mental health.

education – The level of education an individual holds, with higher educational attainment, relates to better levels of health. Low literacy skills are linked to more insecure employment prospects, lower access to health services and more risky health-related behaviours.

employment/working conditions – The nature and security of work available to an individual, with employed people generally healthier than the unemployed. Health is also influenced by specific conditions of employment, including remuneration, with certain types of workers (e.g. white-collar professionals) enjoying healthier work environments than others (e.g. non-unionized sweatshop workers). The degree of control an individual has over his/her employment conditions is also related to health status in terms of work-related stress.

physical environment – The natural and human-made environments in which an individual lives is directly related to health. Clean air and water, safe and warm housing, safe working conditions, fertile soil, adequate fuel supplies, and well-developed community structures all contribute to good health.

personal health practices and coping skills – The types of behaviour that individuals engage in are important factors in determining health status. This include diet, smoking and drinking habits, hygiene, physical exercise and engagement in risk behaviours (e.g. sexual practices, dangerous sports). Coping skills refers to the ability to develop normal social relationships and to deal with life stresses and challenges.

healthy child development – The physical and mental experiences of childhood influence the health of an individual as an adult. These include receiving basic needs such as food, education and clothing, as well as emotional nurturing.

biology and genetic endowment – The genetic makeup of an individual, as inherited from parents, is a strong determinant of health. This is most directly relevant in relation to genetically inherited disorders (e.g. sickle cell disease) but also to inherited physical features that may be related indirectly to health in later life (e.g. obesity).

Box 6.1 continued

health services – The degree of access by an individual to effective health services is related to level of health in terms of the prevention of disease, receiving appropriate treatments and obtaining health promotion messages.

gender – The profile of diseases and conditions differs between men and women at different ages. This may be due to differences in income levels, types of employment, ways of coping with mental stress, roles in reproduction, and social attitudes and treatment.

culture – The traditions, beliefs, value systems and moral ethics of a society influence the health of individuals and population groups. This is manifested, for example through certain cultural practices, treatment of individuals or groups, and dietary habits.

Source: Based on Health Canada (2000), 'What is the population health approach?' <www.hc.sc.gc.ca/hppb/phdd/approach/index.html>

How is globalization affecting factors that determine human health? To what extent are the determinants of health becoming globalized in themselves? How is globalization affecting health outcomes or status? And to what extent are health outcomes or status becoming globalized in their manifestation?

It is at this juncture that the distinction between internationalization and globalization is helpful for drawing out the particular characteristics of global health. As described in Chapter 3, internationalization describes a process of more intense *crossborder* flows or connections between national domains (countries). People interact more frequently than ever before across national borders but the integrity of the state remains intact. Globalization, in contrast, describes a process whereby territorial space, including national borders, become relatively less important and, in some cases, irrelevant because of *transborder* flows of people, goods and services, capital and ideas. New forms of social space may emerge that redefine our sense of territory or create human relationships that are deterritorialized.

This distinction, in turn, helps us to draw more precise boundaries around the emerging concept of global health. In many cases, health issues described as 'global' in the existing literature can be more accurately seen as 'international'. The growing trade in health services is, strictly speaking, within the realm of international health because it concerns the flow of health professionals, services and patients across national borders. The state remains intact because of relatively effective means of regulating these flows. Similarly, the trade in pharmaceuticals can be described as international rather than global because of the generally close national regulation of imports and exports. However, the unregulated flow of such goods and services across borders through, for example, the internet[1] or illicit channels can be seen as global health because of the limited ability of national authorities to control them. National borders are rendered irrelevant, to some degree, in such transactions.

Another useful contrast is the health consequences arising from the flow of people across national borders. The increased flow of tourists, business people, students and other documented migrants give rise to international health issues as long as national authorities have the ability to regulate their movement (and hence their health needs). The enforcement of the WHO's International Health Regulations (IHR) and screening by health officials for certain conditions, albeit controversially perhaps, at ports of entry are examples of such measures. Admittedly, the sheer volume of population mobility increasingly brings into question the logistical capacity for states to carry out such controls effectively. In principle, however, it is possible with sufficient resources and appropriate rules and regulations to reduce crossborder health risks.

The situation becomes very different where health risks cannot be effectively controlled at ports of entry, either because the condition is not detectable or people are not crossing borders through legitimate routes. The former draws attention to the important point that many health conditions cannot be excluded through screening at national borders. Historically, infectious diseases have been the focus of such efforts, with some success, through requirements for vaccination certificates (as for yellow fever) or diagnostic screening (such as for tuberculosis). More controversially, evidence of disease-free status can be required by some governments as a precondition for entry, as in the case of HIV/AIDS. It remains debatable whether some of these requirements are necessary, clinically effective or ethical. Nonetheless, they are used. For other conditions, incubation periods may mean a person does not display observable signs of disease at the time of travelling but may pose a public health risk later on. Or they may pose a risk during transit. Still more problematic is the growing numbers of undocumented migrants whose movements undermine the relevance of national borders. The health issues related to undocumented migrants is a complex challenge, with the tendency so far to view the issue primarily in terms of asylum and immigration policy. Yet the health needs of such migrants, and the communities they move among prior to, during and after travelling all have relevance to global health (Collin and Lee 2003).

A third example is the health impacts of intensifying flows of cultural goods which have both international and global dimensions. As discussed in Chapter 5, world imports of cultural goods rose from US$47.5 billion in 1980 to US$213.7 billion in 1998 (UNESCO 2000). To a large extent, such goods are subject to the control of national authorities who may regulate their form or content to protect public interests in terms of standards of decency, truthfulness, appropriateness to local cultures, or intellectual property. In a growing number of ways, cultural goods can circumvent national control through the technologies used (for example, the internet or satellite television), or innovative forms of marketing and advertising, such as product placement and brand stretching, that can elude regulation. The health consequences arising from such practices, such as influences on lifestyle and health-seeking behaviours, can be described as global.

In summary, global health concerns the ways in which globalization is impacting on both the determinants of health and health outcomes. The degree to which a health determinant or outcome is considered 'global' is usefully understood in relative terms. Where a national government can assert relative control over crossborder flows that impact on the health of the population within its territorial boundaries, the term international health is more accurate. Where there is an erosion of that control by transborder flows that undermine, or even disregard territorial space, the term global health is more appropriate. It is not simply that health determinants and their consequences spill over national borders. It is the degree to which state institutions can manage such spillovers effectively. This book has explored a wide range of ways that globalization is creating spillovers that cannot be effectively controlled and managed by the state. It is from this conceptual starting point that practical action can begin to be built.

6.3   The changing nature of health inequalities

The accidental globalization of the late 20th century has loaded some of us with every comfort. Now it's the turn of the five billion others.
       Diane Coyle, Presenter, 'Analysis: Globalising Doom' (2001)

If we look at health worldwide as a broad canvas, the improvements achieved during the second half of the twentieth century are indisputably impressive. Between 1950 and 1999 average life expectancy at birth increased from 46 to 64 years (WHO 1999c), or four months each year since 1970 (World Bank 2001). Under-five mortality rates declined from 16 per cent in the 1960s to 8 per cent during the 1990s (Jha and Mills 2002), and infant mortality dropped 11 per cent in the developing world since 1990 (World Bank 2001). This rate of progress has been far greater than corresponding changes in health status in Europe and North America during the nineteenth and early twentieth centuries. Such statistics paint an impressive picture of government effort, philanthropic generosity, scientific advancement and international cooperation.

The danger of such a broad perspective, however, is that aggregate data average out significant and persistent health inequalities within and across countries. National health data, taken as a whole or aggregated together regionally and internationally, conceal more worrying patterns and trends that suggest all is not well in global health terms. In recent years, greater attention to these inequalities has been achieved. Both the political left and right acknowledge that important health challenges remain to be addressed worldwide. The causes of these problems, how they can be tackled and, in relation to this book, what role globalization plays in both of these questions, remain highly contested.

This book argues that the relationship between current forms of globalization, inequality and health is an important feature of the emerging order that deserves more concerted attention. The precise cause–effect relationship among the three variables remains disputed. It is widely accepted that absolute and relative inequalities of various kinds contribute to poorer health. In general, the populations of wealthier countries are healthier than populations in poorer countries:

- Of the 56 million deaths worldwide each year, 80 per cent occur in poor regions.
- 90 per cent of the global burden of disease is carried by the developing world, which has access to 10 per cent of the world's resources for health.
- Seven out of ten deaths in children under five years occur in low-income countries.
- Among 191 countries, Japan enjoys the longest life expectancy at 74.5 years while Sierra Leone has the lowest at 26 years (WHO 2000).

- In the UK the median age at death is 77 years compared to two years in Guinea (Pimentel Simbulan 1999)
- Between 1990 and 1999 child mortality increased in sub-Saharan Africa from 155 to 161 per 1000 (World Bank 2001).
- Maternal mortality ranges from six per 100,000 in Australia to 1800 per 100,000 in Sierra Leone (Sen and Bonita 2000).
- One-tenth of deaths in the developing world (1.6 million) are caused by conditions (measles, tetanus, diphtheria) routinely vaccinated for in high-income countries (Jha and Mills 2002: 5).

There is also convincing evidence that the more advantaged individuals and population groups within a given country tend to enjoy better health than the disadvantaged:

- In Peru rates of underweight and stunting among the poorest 20 per cent is about five times that of the richest 20 per cent (Wagstaff and Watanabe 2000).
- In the US, the life expectancy at birth of African-American males is up to 20 years less than for white males (Murray et al. 1994).
- In Mali, 67 per cent of children in the highest quintile of family income receive immunizations for diphtheria, pertussis and tetanus (DPT), compared with only 17 per cent in the lowest quintile (Jha and Mills 2002).
- In India the prevalence of tuberculosis, childhood mortality and tobacco use is three times higher among the lowest income groups than among the highest (Jha and Mills 2002).
- In the Ukraine, almost twice as many women (43 per cent) as men (25 per cent) rate their health as poor, with women in rural areas particularly at risk (Gilmore et al. 2002).

It is thus widely recognized that inequalities within and across countries remain a key health challenge that deserves direct and prolonged policy effort.

What is not so well understood, and rather more disputed, is how globalization impacts on the health and inequality equation (see Figure 6.1). To what extent is globalization contributing to increased inequalities in terms of socioeconomic status, employment conditions, education and so on (arrow [a])? The balance of available data focuses on socioeconomic status. While the precise relationship between globalization and socioeconomic status remains contested (Dollar and Kraay 2000; Weisbrot et al. 2001), with some arguing that it is *more* globalization, not *less*, that is needed to speed the process of economic growth and ultimately improve standards of living for all (Feachem 2001), the existing evidence strongly suggests that current forms of globalization are contributing to widening inequalities in wealth (UNDP 1999). As described in Chapter 3, these inequalities are both stark and unprecedented, with the income of the richest 1 per cent of the world's population now equivalent to the poorest 57 per cent (Milanovic 2002). Although the proportion of the world's population living in poverty has declined from 28 per cent in 1987 to 23 per cent in 1998, the absolute number of poor has increased because of population growth. According to the World Bank (2001), 1.3 billion people live in extreme economic poverty defined as less than US$1 per day (1993 purchasing power parity), with women accounting for 70 per cent. More than three billion live on less than US$2 per day. The 'poorest billion' are distributed widely across Latin America, Africa and Asia, but tend to be concentrated in certain regions. India leads with 400 million of the world's poor, followed by China with 235 million. In sub-Saharan Africa, there are ten countries where 50 per cent or more of the population lives on less than US$1 per day (Jha and Mills 2002). Overall, as the UNDP (1999) reports, 'the accelerating process of globalization is expanding global opportunities without distributing them equitably. The playing fields of globalization more often than not slope against the interest of poor people and countries.'

As well as socioeconomic status, an understanding of the link between globalization and inequality requires recognition of other factors that shape the emerging global 'pecking order' and determine

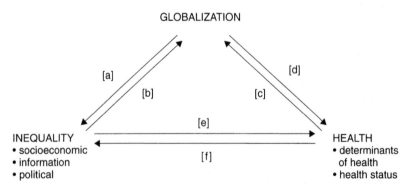

Figure 6.1   The relationship between globalization, inequality and health

where one is located in it. Foremost are the stark inequalities of access to the information and communication technologies (ICTs) that drive and define globalization. About 5 per cent of the world's population (332 million) uses the internet, 88 per cent of whom live in high-income countries. While half of the world's population has never made a telephone call, the Manhattan district of New York has more telephone lines than the whole of Africa (UNDP 1999). The situation in Africa is especially problematic, with over 12 per cent of the world's population yet only 2 per cent of telephone lines (NUA 1998). In the health field, there are high hopes that telemedicine[2] will be an important means of facilitating health development. Telemedicine refers to the use of ICTs to provide medical care where the provider is far from the patient. This can range from telephone contact between patient and provider, exchange of complex information and images, and even remote surgical or diagnostic procedures. In an effort to address the so-called 'digital divide', UN Secretary-General Kofi Annan announced the WHO-led Health InterNetwork project in 2000 aimed at strengthening public health systems through timely, relevant and high-quality health information through an internet portal, as well as improve communication and networking. Similarly, a three-year initiative began in January 2002 by WHO and the world's six biggest medical journal publishers to reduce 'the health information gap between rich and poor countries'. The initiative allows around 100 low- and middle-income countries to gain electronic access to almost 1000 of the world's leading medical and scientific journals free or at reduced rates (WHO 2001). Projects such as these, aimed at levelling the playing field between the information 'rich' and 'poor' will be an essential component of tackling inequalities in health.

Another important form of inequality, one that may prove most intransigent, is the lack of sufficient voice by certain population groups in global decision making. Ultimately, inequality in a globalizing world is about inequalities in political power. There is strong feeling, backed by growing evidence, that the emerging global order is an exclusive one in terms of who participates in decision making and who is excluded. Core global institutions, such as the WTO, World Bank and IMF, have all been criticized for their dominance by the interests of big business and big government (that is, of high-income countries). For example, the presidency of the World Bank is always held by a US citizen as per political custom, while the head of the IMF is always a European. More structural is the balance of nationalities among their staff, the venues chosen for their major meetings, their financing, and their voting systems. Perhaps most fundamentally, their strong ideological underpinnings in neoliberalism, particular organizational cultures, and resultant 'rules of the game' narrow the range of perspectives entertained within them and close off certain avenues of policy debate. Other institutional mechanisms underpinning globalization that have arisen in recent decades, notably the World Economic Forum and Group of Eight countries, similarly show limited signs of creating more democratic forms of participation.

It is unclear how international health organizations fit into this emerging order. The universal membership of WHO, with its UN-based one-state, one-vote system, makes it more democratic in principle than, for example, the World Bank. Some of the more recent forms of global health cooperation, such as the Global Fund to Fight AIDS, Tuberculosis and Malaria, has sought to include broad representation in its governance (see Box 5.3). Nonetheless, as described in Chapter 5, the setting of international and global health policies have been far from a rational process. How health priorities are set at various levels of policy making from the local to the global are oftentimes shaped by dominant interests able to disproportionately influence the policy agenda. In a system where 'the squeaky wheel gets the oil', those without sufficient financial, intellectual and political resources to voice their health needs find themselves at a disadvantage.

As well as its direct impact on inequalities (Figure 6.1 arrow [a]), which have health consequences (arrow [e]), there is a need to better understand how globalization affects health and, in turn, inequalities (arrows [d] and [f]). This book has begun to explore some of these cause–effect links between globalization and health, bearing in mind that the empirical evidence currently available is variable and limited. In addition, recalling the health determinants described in Box 6.1, we can see that it is a major analytical challenge to separate out what are closely interrelated factors at play. Yet, the examples provided in this book suggest many avenues to explore (Box 6.2).

Notably, it is important to recognize that health impacts from globalization do not necessarily conform to national boundaries. As Chapter 3 concludes, globalization is creating new 'populations' that require identification and analyses, populations that (a) do not conform to state-defined territorial boundaries; and (b) may not even be territorially defined. It is along these parameters that new patterns of health and disease, including inequalities in health, may be emerging. Although the statecentric nature of available health data[3] makes this difficult to measure, it is possible to begin identifying what these populations are, and their health needs, on the basis of their position in the emerging global order. For example, undocumented migrants are at particular risk of infectious disease, violence and injury, and are less likely to gain access to health services. Similarly, unskilled and non-unionized workers suffer from a greater incidence of occupational diseases because of weaker health and safety protection and, hence, greater exposure to risky environments. The middle class in urban areas across many countries are experiencing a rising incidence of being overweight and obese because of rising incomes, exposure to the marketing of consumer goods, and changing diets and lifestyles. Populations living at altitudes near sea level are at greater risk in future of flooding and severe weather, and hence waterborne diseases, due to global climate change. In short, we need to identify and understand better how globalization is creating additional patterns of health inequality that may remain hidden by aggregated national data. What defines the health needs of these population groups is not their territorial location but their 'place' in the emerging global order, part of what Murphy (2000) calls the 'new inequality'.

Finally, the imperative for understanding and addressing the link between inequality and health is given more political momentum by the impact that they can have on globalization itself (Figure 6.1 arrows [b] and [c]). As shown by Working Group 5 of the Commission on Macroeconomics and Health, which considered the challenge of improving health outcomes of the poor, inequalities contribute to poor health (Jha and Mills 2002). Poor health, in turn, is a significant drain on a society's capacity to develop economically. Globally, health inequalities can contribute to greater social and economic instability, undermining the capacity of states and preventing them from participating in the global economy (Price-Smith 2002). Perhaps most starkly, health inequalities create consequences far beyond the individuals and communities worst affected by them. Would HIV/AIDS have spread as quickly in a more equitable world? Would multidrug resistant tuberculosis (MDRTB) have emerged and spread if it was not predominantly a disease of the poor? The resources needed to address the health needs of the world's poor are recognized as substantial (US$40–56 billion in increased annual expenditure by 2015). The rationale for providing them, in this sense, is a shared interest in creating an inclusive form of globalization of shared rights and responsibilities.

6.4   Health and the sustainability of globalization

The global economy we are creating can ... only massively increase environmental destruction – not only by increasing its impact on an environment that cannot sustain the present impact but also by eliminating regulations designed to contain this impact ...

Goldsmith (1996: 91)

For every person in the world to reach US levels of consumption with existing technology would require four more planet earths.

Professor E. O. Wilson, Harvard University, as quoted in Johnston (2001)

The health consequences of global environmental change have only been touched upon in this introductory text to give a sense of the intertwining of fates between the natural world and human societies. The concept of *sustainability* lies at the heart of this relationship. Human impacts on the natural environment, along with the impacts of other animal species, have occurred throughout history. What is profoundly different, as accumulating evidence indicates, is the rate and degree of these impacts, many of which may be irreversible. According to the Worldwide Fund for Nature's Living Planet Index (WWF 2002),

The global ecological footprint has grown from about 70% of the planet's biological capacity in 1961 to about 120% of its biological capacity in 1999. Furthermore, future projections based on likely scenarios of population growth, economic development and technological change, show that humanity's footprint is likely to grow to about 180% to 220% of the Earth's biological capacity by the year 2050. Of course, it is very unlikely that the Earth would be able to run an ecological overdraft for another 50 years without some severe ecological backlashes undermining future population and economic growth.

The long-term survival of the human species depends on whether we can reverse these alarming trends by learning how to use the resources available to us in ways, and at rates, that allow them to be regenerated. The erosion of the earth's 'natural capital'[4] and destruction of the earth's biosystems, to the extent that human and other life cannot be sustained, is clearly the ultimate threat to human health.

Yet the evidence reviewed briefly in this book shows that we are far from learning this lesson. The global picture is bleak because of profound inequalities in responsibility for these trends. The five billion people living in the developing world have an ecological footprint of 2.5 acres per person, compared with around 24 acres per person for the US (Johnston 2001). To the extent that current forms of globalization are encouraging the integration of the developing world into a global political economy, defined by modes of production and levels of consumption that are environmentally unsustainable, these trends will worsen. Other policies associated with globalization, such as the privatization of clean water supplies and assertion of intellectual property rights over natural life forms (e.g. indigenous plants, genetic codes) underpins this commodification of the natural environment within a global economy.

Changing patterns of health and disease provide vital evidence of the trajectory we are currently following, and can serve as a touchstone for the sustainability of current globalization practices. The damage to the ozone layer so far has coincided with a marked rise in the incidence of skin cancers (Friends of the Earth 2001). Extreme weather patterns have increased in intensity, resulting in such threats to health as floods, increased disease vectors (for example mosquitoes, rodents) and reduced food production (McMichael and Haines 1997). The pollution of clean water supplies is accompanied by growing rates of waterborne diseases. Intense farming methods by an increasingly globalized agro-industrial complex are creating transborder foodborne risks, as well as dietary shifts towards the overconsumption of fats, salt and sugar. The loss of biodiversity is closing down possible avenues for new treatments and therapies from animal species and natural compounds. In short, the status of human health is a key indicator of the health of the planet as a whole. The two are inextricably intertwined, with environmental sustainability a critical prerequisite to the long-term survival of the human species.

As well as sustainability in terms of the natural environment, globalization raises fundamental challenges for building sustainable social environments. To what extent can societies – where globalization is contributing to widening socioeconomic inequalities, weakened social policies, and rapid changes to established social structures – achieve peace and stability, ensure functioning economies, and build social cohesion? The concept of social sustainability is a variably defined but increasingly recognized one that focuses on the importance of building 'social capital'[5] as part of sustainable development. The principles behind social sustainability are broadly agreed as being sensitive to the needs of vulnerable groups, addressing socioeconomic inequalities, encouraging the participation of relevant stakeholders in decision making, and providing support for building social capital (Polèse and Stren 2000).

Attention to the social consequences of globalization, including its health impacts, have received growing attention. It is recognized that the sustainability of globalization depends much on its capacity to create socially sustainable environments. In South-East Asia, the economic crisis of the late 1990s following rapid growth in the 1980s, brought forward already simmering tensions between 'haves' and 'have nots'. In Indonesia, the situation led to widespread rioting and ultimately to political change with the fall of the Suharto regime in May 1998. The integrated nature of the global economy spread the crisis far and wide to Latin America where countries such as Peru, Argentina, Colombia and Mexico have seen their economies face near collapse. The contagion effect also reached eastern Europe where the 'emerging' economies have struggled since the end of the Cold War. Even in the US, which was relatively unaffected by the global economic crisis of the late 1990s, there are worrying signs. Hutton (2003) describes the US, the most unequal society in the world, as a new feudalism whereby an elite aristocracy sits in sharp contrast atop a poor majority. This, he warns, will lead to internal political and social instability in future which will undermine the country's dominant position. The terrorist attacks of 11 September 2001, and the financial scandals in 2002 involving major corporations, notably Enron and WorldCom, have contributed further to global political and economic instability. These events have shaken confidence that economic globalization will necessarily lead to a bright and shining future. Indeed, far greater attention to the internal weaknesses of the system that threaten social sustainability is recognized, challenges that are discussed below in relation to global governance.

In summary, the concept of sustainability is central to negotiating the links between globalization and human health. It is clear that our individual and collective health is directly dependent on achieving more environmentally sustainable forms of globalization than currently exist. Health can serve as a clear measure of the extent to which this is achieved. Equally relevant is the concept of social sustainability in terms of the quality of values, institutional structures, and formal/informal interactions that help bind a population group together as a collective entity. This book suggests that globalization is pulling in different directions, in some cases bringing communities closer together through shared values and interests, in other ways undermining the social fabric of many communities. Along with preserving the integrity of the natural environment, social sustainability will also be a key determinant of the long-term success of globalization. Again the health sector offers the means of building this foundation, as well as important lessons for reflecting on its effective achievement.

6.5   Good governance for global health

> *Do we shape it or does it shape us? Do we master it, or do we let it overwhelm us? That's the sole key to politics in the modern world: how to manage change. Resist it: futile; let it happen: dangerous. So – the third way – manage it.*

> UK Prime Minister Tony Blair (2000)

Throughout this book, the need to rethink many of the rules and institutions concerned with health has been touched upon. The prospect of reforming and perhaps redefining health governance at various levels, from the local to the global, along with governance of other sectors that impact on the determinants of health, is clearly a daunting one. The task before us is monumental, the barriers to change are seemingly insurmountable, yet the case for change seems compelling. In this concluding chapter of an introductory book, we can only begin to scratch the surface in setting out the challenge at hand, let alone put forward emerging ideas to inform practice. Detailed discussion of the definition of global governance, and the particular policy instruments and institutional structures needed to address specific health issues is beyond the scope of this book, although a good start in thinking about such needs is provided in an accompanying volume, *Health Impacts of Globalization: Towards Global Governance* (2002).

In setting out the main challenges, it is useful to briefly define what we mean by global governance and, in particular, global health governance. A broad definition of governance, offered by the Commission on Global Governance (1995: 2), and one that fits well with the challenges of global health is:

> the sum of the ways individuals and institutions, public and private, manage their common affairs. It is a continuing process through which conflicting or diverse interests may be accommodated and

co-operative action may be taken. It includes formal institutions and regimes, empowered to enforce compliance, as well as informal arrangements that people and institutions either have agreed to or perceive to be in their interest.

The important aspects of this definition are that there are agreed rules governing relationships among individuals and institutions, that these rules facilitate the pursuit of common interests, and that there is a diversity of individuals and institutions involved both formally and informally. Global governance, in turn, concerns governance for the purpose of managing those issues of a global nature, that is, issues involving causes and effects that spill over and even ignore state boundaries to the extent that governments alone are unable to control them effectively (see Section 6.2).

Applied to health, we can see that global governance raises a number of important challenges that have so far only begun to be explored. First, we are in the midst of stumbling from a focus on international to global health governance. The former is focused on national governments and, collectively, intergovernmental organizations such as WHO which work through state institutions to cooperate on health determinants and outcomes that cross national borders. The International Health Regulations administered by WHO are a prime example. Global health governance (GHG), in contrast, concerns cooperation among state and non-state actors to address issues of a transborder nature. While GHG is a nascent form of governance, important examples include the Framework Convention on Tobacco Control (see below), and Global Fund to Fight HIV/AIDS, Tuberculosis and Malaria (see Box 5.3).

The creation of agreed forms of governance that include the diversity of individuals and institutions concerned with global health is a major challenge. In broad terms, institutions can be categorized as falling into three overlapping spheres: state, market and civil society (Figure 6.2). The spheres overlap because some institutions may contribute to more than one sphere, for example, autonomous hospitals (state–market), industry associations (market–civil society) and primary care groups (civil society–state). But they are also depicted as overlapping because of their mutual interdependence. In any society, an imbalance in power of any one of these spheres can lead to the unchecked abuse of that power. As Sen (2000) describes, the 'role of institutions has to be assessed in terms of the "countervailing power" they exercise over one another. Asymmetric power in one domain can be checked in a different configuration of forces in another domain.'

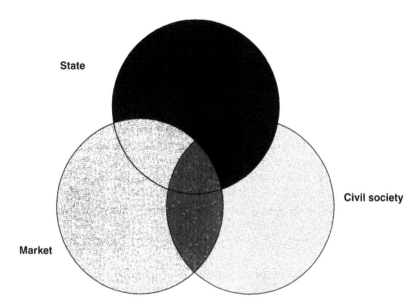

Figure 6.2   The overlapping spheres of the state, market and civil society

The balance of power among these three spheres, and the rules governing the exercise of that power, lie at the heart of emerging forms of global health governance. In terms of governance of globalization in general, many argue that the balance of power is skewed, either in terms of favouring the market over the state and civil society, or in favouring certain states, markets and civil society groups. Perhaps most visibly are supporters of the so-called 'anti-globalization' movement which points to the private sector and, in particular, TNCs seen to increasingly 'rule the world' (Korten 2001). Put rather starkly by Corporate Watch, 'As we move into a new millennium, "We the Peoples" of the United Nations are asking a momentous question: Will corporations rule the world or will they be subordinated by governments and civil society to the universal values of human rights, labor rights and environmental rights' (Bruno and Karliner 2000)? In the health sector, there are concerns that health-related TNCs in the pharmaceutical, food and service industries enjoy a disproportionate influence over the rules defining GHG and how they are applied.

For others, the present distortions in global governance bring together big government and big business, and the institutions that favour their interests. For many working in local communities throughout the developing world, for example, at the coalface of 'adjustment' or 'transition' towards a global political economy, the 'axis of evil' is seen as the triumvirate of the World Bank, IMF and WTO. Their power, backed by the US and other Western governments, and that of other institutions of the so-called Washington Consensus, to pressure the less powerful to adopt 'one size fits all' policies, is challenged both on ethical and democratic grounds, as well as empirical evidence of the negative social consequences in many countries. This discomfort at the blunt realities of globalization has been expressed, not only by anti-globalization campaigners, but by prominent establishment figures such as George Soros (2002) and former chief economist for the World Bank Joseph Stiglitz (Stiglitz 1998). In global health, the marked increase in the World Bank's role in health development since the early 1980s has been seen as subsuming the health sector within its broader neoliberal agenda.

Still others are concerned with imbalances in power that run within and across state and nonstate actors, manifested in the inequalities described in Section 6.3. A number of international relations scholars map out this transnational asymmetry in terms of an emerging global elite, able to set and control the rules of the globalization game to their advantage. Cox (1987), for example, uses the term 'managerial transnational class', van der Pijl (1989) identifies an 'Atlantic ruling class', and Falk (1999) speaks of 'predatory globalization' dominated by global capital and governments. While the cast of characters varies somewhat in each case, notably who gets to play the villain, they share a perspective that the dividing lines of power are being redefined by the transborder nature of globalization. The proliferation of global public–private partnerships in health, bringing together diverse groups of stakeholders across the spheres of the state, market and civil society illustrates this trend.

However one sees the precise balance of power in current forms of globalization, it is widely perceived that there are asymmetries in its governance. These asymmetries mean insufficient checks and balances in the system, creating risks not only to those less powerful but to globalization as a whole. While some believe that the whole globalization project per se should be aborted, most seek to rebalance existing asymmetries through new forms of global governance. In the United States, America's fourth wealthiest man, Warren Buffet, has founded a pressure group to oppose the elimination of taxes on capital gains and inherited wealth, given his concerns about the long-term consequences of the widening gap between rich and poor in the US. As Hutton (2003) describes,

> Just as it would be absurd to select the US Olympics team for 2020 from the children of the winners of the Olympics in 2000, so it is wrong to construct a society whose likely leaders tomorrow – given the advantages that wealth confers – will be the children of today's wealthy. This offends not merely the values of democracy and equality of opportunity on which the US is constructed, but will be economically disastrous.

Within the financial sector, the volatility of capital markets has led to high-level efforts to strengthen global economic governance by, for example, creating 'speed bumps' to prevent speculative trading.[6] More broadly, changes to the policy priorities of the World Bank, under President James Wolfensohn, have given stronger emphasis to the social sectors and poverty alleviation. In the wake of mass demonstrations at major international meetings, there has been greater recognition of the need for more transparency and wider participation in the WTO, World Bank and IMF. Effective campaigns by global civil society have contributed to putting debt relief, child labour and other social issues onto the policy agendas of major international organizations. Finally, there has been a new generation of philanthropists who seek to 'make a difference' and large businesses are awash with corporate social responsibility initiatives.

The health community has also been grappling with the challenges of reforming existing institutions, and creating new forms of governance, to meet changing health needs amidst globalization. It is a transition fraught with different understandings about the priorities faced, and diverse perspectives on what is to be achieved. The establishment of the main pillars of international health cooperation were historically spurred by major events – epidemics of infectious disease led to the International Sanitary Conferences; the First World War and the influenza pandemic of 1918–19 contributed to the creation of the Health Organization of the League of Nations; and the lessons from the Second World War led to the establishment of WHO. While there has not been a 'defining moment' comparable to the scale of these events so far, a constellation of worrying developments is steadily pushing the agenda forward. These include newly emerging diseases notably the HIV/AIDS pandemic, the re-emergence of diseases such as tuberculosis and malaria, the continued spread of antimicrobial resistance, and the spectre of large-scale biological and chemical weapons. Furthermore, there is a sense that health is clearly a common and universal good, and that there is a shared interest in fostering cooperation. Finally, in the highly charged political environments within which anti-globalization protests, G8 summits, and trade negotiations take place, health is seen as relatively neutral ground where divergent interests can come together for a common good.

It is for these reasons that the health sector has been the subject of a wide range of nascent forms of global governance. Most have yet to be documented in detail, let alone critically analysed in terms of their characteristics and effectiveness at meeting health needs. It is worth mentioning three of these developments in order to identify their distinct nature, and the governance challenges they are seeking to address.

6.5.1 *Framework Convention on Tobacco Control*

In 1999 the WHA unanimously adopted Resolution 52.18 to initiate a two-step process for negotiating a Framework Convention on Tobacco Control (FCTC). Working groups began to establish the technical foundations of such an agreement, followed by the establishment of an Intergovernmental Negotiating Body (INB) to undertake rounds of detailed negotiations among WHO member states. The scale of member state involvement has been impressive,[7] triggering intersectoral discussions on tobacco issues within countries, and regular interministerial consultations across countries. An additional objective of WHO was to improve coordination and cooperation across UN agencies. A key step was the establishment of an Ad Hoc Inter-Agency Task Force on Tobacco Control in 1999 under the leadership of WHO. This replaced the previous focal point in the UN, the UN Conference on Trade and Development (UNCTAD), which had 'opened the door to tobacco industry influence throughout the UN' (Committee of Experts 2000). Engaging the World Bank in tobacco control issues was particularly important in countering often cited arguments about the economic benefits of tobacco (Jha and Chaloupka 2000).

Notable, in terms of proto forms of global governance, were efforts within the FCTC negotiation process to more actively involve actors traditionally excluded from the state-centric deliberations of WHO. In public hearings held by WHO in October 2000, the first of their kind, over 500 written submissions were received, and 144 organizations provided oral testimony during the two-day hearing encompassing TTCs, state tobacco companies and producer organizations, public health organizations, women's groups and research institutions (WHO 2000a). WHO did not seek to engage with the tobacco industry, understandably in light of compelling evidence of ongoing industry tactics to undermine the organization and covertly pressure individual member state delegations (Brundtland 2000b). In other spheres, however, WHO was not reluctant to engage with the private sector. WHO is committed to exploring the role of nicotine replacement therapy in smoking cessation programmes including cooperation with pharmaceutical companies. For World No Tobacco Day 2000, with the theme of smoking cessation, marketing expertise and financial assistance were accepted from the pharmaceutical industry. More specifically, two industry associations have worked with WHO on this issue. A representative of the World Self-Medication Industry (WSMI) sat on the Policy and Strategy Advisory Committee (PSAC), an advisory committee that reported to WHO Director General Gro Harlem Brundtland on tobacco control between 1999 and May 2001. Collaborative activities with the International Federation of Pharmaceutical Manufacturers Association (IFPMA) was also developed.

Another way of widening participation was through WHO provisions for officially recognizing NGOs. 'Official Relations' is a status achieved through a multi-year process by international health-related NGOs, usually international federations of national and regional professional NGOs. There are currently 193 NGOs in Official Relations with WHO, entitling them to observe proceedings and to 'make a statement of an expository nature' at the invitation of the chair (WHO 2000b), generally restricted to a short period at the end of a session. NGOs not in official relations must find a sponsoring organization to enter and observe a formal meeting, and are barred from making statements in the name of their organization. In order to contribute more fully to the FCTC process, NGOs sought to ease these stipulations, supported by a number of member states, notably Canada. Following an open consultation, member states approved recommendations that the process of accreditation should be accelerated and that NGOs in official relations have access to open working groups. It was later agreed that NGOs could be given provisional 'Official Relations' status to enable their participation in the FCTC process.

Perhaps more important than participating formally in negotiations, NGOs were encouraged to play a diverse range of supporting roles. Prominent among these was an educative function, with NGOs organizing seminars and briefings for delegates on diverse technical aspects of the proposed Convention. Outside of negotiations, lobbying activities were extensive through discussions with governments, letter-writing to delegates and heads of state, advocacy campaigns, press conferences, and the distribution of published materials. The NGOs were also able to use their presence to act as a public health conscience during proceedings, lauding some member states for their supportive interventions, chastising others for their obstructionist positions. Daily newsletters, produced and distributed at negotiations and worldwide via the internet were an important part of this work.

Finally, the composition of member state delegates is worth noting. One way tobacco companies secured participation in the FCTC process was by serving on delegations, the composition of which is beyond WHO jurisdiction. One example is Turkey whose delegation to the negotiations included Oktay Önderer, the Deputy Director General of TEKEL, the state tobacco monopoly (WHO 1999b, 2000a). BAT is reported to have successively pressed representatives of China's state tobacco company to ensure their inclusion in the Chinese delegation, while a spokesman for Japan Tobacco/R J Reynolds asserted that the company had successfully made its case against the FCTC in Russia, Romania and Turkey (Loewenberg 2000). At the same time, however, prominent tobacco control advocates participated in negotiations from within national delegations, including John Kapito, Margaretha Haglund and Luc Joossens for Malawi, Sweden and Belgium respectively (WHO 2000a).

Overall, the FCTC process is an interesting one for those interested in following emerging forms of governance for global health.[8] WHO describes the rapid increase in the use of tobacco worldwide as a 'global public health emergency', and the FCTC is intended to be a response to the global nature of the issue. As an intergovernmental treaty signed in 2003, it sets out a regulatory framework for member states to develop national level legislation and regulation for tobacco control. The involvement of non-state actors in the negotiating process and, equally importantly, implementation of the treaty, will strongly determine the extent to which it will create a form of governance that will effectively address factors that do not respect national boundaries.

6.5.2   *International Women's Health Coalition*

While the FCTC can be seen as ostensibly an intergovernmental process with important inputs from non-state actors, the International

Women's Health Coalition (IWHC) is a social movement defined by non-state actors working 'to generate health and population policies, programs, and funding that promote and protect the rights and health of girls and women worldwide, particularly in Africa, Asia, Latin America and countries in postsocialist transition' (IWHC 2002). The origins of the women's health movement can be traced to the US where women's groups, such as the National Women's Health Network (NWHN) and Boston Women's Health Book Collective (publishers of *Our Bodies, Ourselves*), began campaigning in the 1970s for greater recognition and sensitivity to the particular health needs of women. The creation of the Office of Women's Health in the US National Institutes of Health in 1990 gave formal recognition to 'women's health' but it remained narrowly biomedical in its focus on obstetrics and gynaecology. Women's groups continue to campaign for women's health throughout the lifespan.

The extension of the women's health movement to the global level was boosted by two major meetings of feminist groups held in 1977 in Amsterdam and Paris. Attended by hundreds of women, mainly from Europe but also other regions of the world, they facilitated the bringing together of issues such as safe abortion, sterilization abuse, domestic violence and access to contraception. The term 'reproductive rights' was first used in the late 1970s by the American group Campaign for Abortion Rights and Against Sterilization Abuse (CARASA), and began to be taken up at international meetings in the early 1980s as an appropriate description of the range of issues being tackled. Examples of abuses began to be documented in the developing world – forced sterilization in India, one-child policy in China, female genital mutilation in parts of Africa – hence broadening the network of organizations coming together under the banner of reproductive rights (Berer 1997).

The International Conference on Population and Development (ICPD) held in Cairo in 1994 showcased the extent to which women's groups around the world had mobilized around reproductive health. Their aim at the conference was to shift public attention from population control, which had dominated previous conferences, to the right of women to reproductive health. For this purpose, the IWHC was formed in the early 1990s as a large, informal coalition of NGOs concerned, not only with women's health, but social and development issues based around the world (Doyal 1996). Its success in achieving a fundamental paradigm shift at the ICPD led it to target other major conferences such as the Fourth World Conference on Women (Beijing 1995) and ICPD Plus Five (1999). While the IWHC has succeeded in organizing itself and creating a solid network of politically active and effective groups, it sees its toughest challenge as achieving the actual implementation of hard-fought agreements in communities around the world (IWHC 2002).

It is perhaps arguable whether the IWHC can be described as a global social movement, in the sense that its formation was the result of bottom–up or 'grassroots globalization'. The initial lead role of women's groups from high-income countries in initiating the movement is clear. There has also been some criticism that the movement remains dominated by the educated middle class across high- and low-income countries, and does not sufficiently represent the everyday reality of many women. However, it would be inaccurate to dismiss the IWHC as one wholly defined by a small elite or one that does not represent the views of a major population group. The IWHC is an illustrative example of the manner in which a non-territorially defined population group, in this case by gender, has come together to assert political power over health issues that cut across national boundaries. It has achieved this by using the technologies of globalization, notably the internet, and by joining together with like-minded groups to build alliances across countries and issue areas. Global social movements have been a major political force within the health field in recent decades, growing in number and organizational strength. By the late 1990s, health groups joined forces with 'anti-globalization' protesters, forming for instance the People's Health Movement (Box 6.2), to reform the emerging order.

6.5.3 *Global Public Health Intelligence Network*

Accurate and timely surveillance and reporting of communicable disease outbreaks is a core function of any effective system of disease prevention, control and treatment. While the International Health Regulations and other agreements require governments to report such outbreaks, systems for doing so are highly variable in capacity from country to country. At the same time, news of reported outbreaks can have serious and sometimes disproportionate economic impacts for the source country, resulting in a degree of reluctance at times by governments to report such information to the international community. Nonetheless, globalization heightens the importance of such information because of increased risks from crossborder and transborder transmission of pathogens.

Box 6.2   The People's Health Movement

The People's Health Movement came together in the late 1990s 'to build a concerted international effort to put the goal of Health for All in its rightful place on the development agenda'. As a loose coalition of like-minded international organizations, NGOs, women's groups, and other civil society groups, the movement aims to put pressure on governments, international organizations and the private sector to ensure that the vision expressed in the Declaration of Alma-Ata is achieved.*

In December 2000 the movement held a People's Health Assembly in Savar, Bangladesh, attended by over 1400 participants from 92 countries. Preparations for the meeting took 18 months in the form of thousands of village meetings, district level workshops and national gatherings. Background papers were prepared on a wide range of topics related to major health issues facing ordinary people around the world. These issues were then discussed at the Assembly. Much attention focused on the implications of multilateral trade agreements under the World Trade Organization for health equity, and the impact of World Bank policies on global health.

At the end of the Assembly, participants formulated and endorsed the People's Charter for Health described as 'the common tool of a worldwide citizen's movement committed to making the Alma-Ata dream a reality'. The Charter states:

> Health is a social, economic and political issue and above all a fundamental human right. Inequality, poverty, exploitation, violence and injustice are at the root of ill-health and the deaths of poor and marginalised people. Health for all means that powerful interests have to be challenged, that globalisation has to be opposed, and that political and economic priorities have to be drastically changed.
>
> This Charter builds on perspectives of people whose voices have rarely been heard before, if at all. It encourages people to develop their own solutions and to hold accountable local authorities, national governments, international organisations and corporations.
>
> Equity, ecologically-sustainable development and peace are at the heart of our vision of a better world – a world in which a healthy life for all is a reality; a world that respects, appreciates and celebrates all life and diversity; a world that enables the flowering of people's talents and abilities to enrich each other; a world in which people's voices guide the decisions that shape our lives. There are more than enough resources to achieve this vision.

Source: The People's Health Movement website, <www.phamovement. org.about.html>

*The International Conference on Primary Health Care, also known as the Alma-Ata Conference, was held by WHO and UNICEF in 1978 in response to

---

Box 6.2   continued

growing concerns over the widespread inequities that existed between health and health care in the industrialized and developing worlds. The conference was preceded by the adoption of the Health for All by the Year 2000 initiative by WHO member states in 1977 which set as a target the achievement by the end of the millennium of a level of health that permits all people to live socially and economically productives lives. The Alma-Ata Conference set out the main strategy for achieving this target, the primary health care approach, which focused on meeting basic health needs through appropriate and affordable means.

The Global Public Health Intelligence Network (GPHIN) is a project created in 1998 by the Laboratory Centre for Disease Control (LCDC) of the Canadian ministry of health, Health Canada, as an early warning, real-time search system that scans the internet for news of infectious disease outbreaks around the world. Working in partnership with WHO, GPHIN is an internet browser that continually scans about 600 international sources for news of outbreaks of 31 communicable diseases, as well as articles about natural disasters and drug-resistant pathogens. As soon as an outbreak is identified, the system notifies the officials at WHO responsible for verifying the information. The website is also limited to a recognized number of public health organizations and professionals to minimize irresponsible or inappropriate use of information (Health Canada 1999). The system currently manages to identify five outbreaks per day on average. It is so far limited to English and French language sources, and to communicable disease surveillance. There are plans to expand searching to all official languages of WHO, and to cover noncommunicable diseases, food and water safety, environmental health risks, and the health impact of natural disasters (Grein et al. 2000).

GPHIN is an interesting example of emerging forms of GHG because of its reliance on both state and non-state sources of information, and its reliance on the internet. Traditionally, communicable disease surveillance has relied on the reports of governments which may be either inaccurate or slow to materialize. This information is usually sent via telephone or facsimile. GPHIN scans a wide range of sources including major news agencies, newspapers, biomedical journals, electronic discussion groups such as ProMed,[9] religious mission networks and NGOs (WHO 1998a). The powerful search engines used by the system to trawl the internet 24 hours a day, provide more rapid acquisition and dissemination of information.

There are many more examples of emerging forms of governance related to global health that deserve greater analytical attention than can be offered here. These include means of interregional cooperation, a plethora of public–private partnerships, new philanthropists, and the negotiation and interpretation of agreements under the WTO. A concerted and comprehensive effort to assess these in detail is urgently needed (Dodgson et al. 2002).

Together, they represent a collective sense that change is needed in the governance of health. Ongoing efforts to reform health systems at the national level continue in countries around the world, facing changing epidemiological and demographic trends, struggling to optimize limited resources, and developing and adopting new interventions. The search to find an appropriate path from international to global health cooperation is, in many ways, an extension of these reform efforts. Indeed, a key message of this book is that the traditional distinction between domestic and global determinants of health cannot be sustained. The neat institutional separation of departments of health, with their collective heads focused on pressing demands at home, and WHO, with its mandate of addressing the health needs of member states, has been revealed as having serious gaps in capacity, authority and responsibility. The issues discussed in this book suggest that health institutions originating in the nineteenth and twentieth centuries must be better equipped to deal effectively with globalization as it is now impacting on health.

Recalling the dimensions of global change that form the conceptual framework of this book, we can summarize the issues that form an emerging agenda for global health governance. First, protecting the territorial integrity of national borders, through such traditional measures as quarantine, *cordon sanitaire* and screening at ports of entry, makes increasingly little sense with the reterritorialization and deterritorialization of many health determinants. Intensified population mobility, illicit activities, climate change, and the internet all challenge the reliance on territorial space as a means of controlling health risks. At the same time, global disease surveillance, wider dissemination of medical research, and capacity to mobilize human and financial resources to tackle health emergencies offer potential health benefits. Just as Christopher Colombus shook prevailing thought by proving that the world was round not flat, our sense of the world since the fifteenth century as one carved up into individual nation-states may need to give way to a paradigmatic shift towards a more holistic notion of the world in its entirety. How do we organize health governance spatially in a manner that effectively captures and manages health determinants and outcomes being changed by globalization?

Second, governance for global health requires timeliness in line with the temporal changes being brought about by globalization. Chapter 4 discusses how globalization is affecting the speed, frequency and duration of many important aspects of our lives. The health consequences are diverse and, in many cases, profound. They range from the rate at which genetic material is passed intergenerationally, to the long-term sustainability of the earth's biosystems. Contemporary health institutions are attuned to certain timescales, dictated by such things as political elections, and budget and planning cycles. Rapid events and long-term changes such as climate change are more difficult to deal with, especially when combined with transborder factors that flow into multiple jurisdictions. How can we design systems of health governance to deal with the temporal changes that globalization is creating?

Finally, global health is not only about being at the right place at the right time. It is also about diverse and competing ideas about the priorities to hand, and the most appropriate and effective means of addressing them. Underpinning those ideas are different values that require suitable venues to mediate among them. The sources of those ideas and values are changing as a consequence of globalization. Multilateral institutions, such as the World Bank, IMF and regional development banks, play a strong role in defining the policy frameworks for economies throughout the world, supported by an army of consultants, research institutions and think tanks. TNCs, and their extended family of suppliers, distributors, and advertising companies influence our individual and collective desires for certain lifestyles. Cultural goods, such as films, television and radio, books, and the mass media, again socialize us through increasingly transborder messages. Civil society groups also encourage us to support certain values as expressed through specific causes or the needs of certain population groups. What systems of health governance do we need to ensure the democratic mediation of competing value systems?

6.6   Conclusions

To the extent to which this book serves as a catalyst for raising questions, and initiating a concerted search for more answers to the challenges posed by globalization for our health, it has served its purpose. It remains an imperfect book. The framework used, focusing on the spatial, cognitive and temporal dimensions of globalization, is a heuristic one for bringing a degree of analytical order to what is a highly complex, multilevelled, multidisciplinary and intersectoral subject. The examples provided scratch the surface of the long list of issues before us – there is so much more to say. In addition, it is easy to slip into 'doom and gloom' mode because bad news sells, and because of the nature of the evidence we have to work with at present, but also because there are worrying things happening. Finally, it is also a subject that is highly contested and thus politically charged in its content and intent. The lines between medical science and global politics are not always sharply defined.

Nonetheless, these challenges lie before us all as globalization continues apace. Do we throw our collective hands in the air and lament that these are forces beyond human control? Or, if controllable, do we rail that we are powerless to change them because the means of control are in the hands of a powerful elite? Or do we look the other way because either globalization or health is a specialist subject that is beyond our personal knowledge and/or experience. It is the intention of this book to encourage at least an engagement with the subject, and to demonstrate that our health as individuals, and the collective health of human populations worldwide, is inextricably bound together. From this starting point, the choices we face can be made clearer.

Key Readings

Farmer P. (2001), *Infections and Inequalities: The Modern Plagues,* 2nd edition (Berkeley: University of California Press).

Garrett L. (2001), *Betrayal of Trust: The Collapse of Global Health* (Oxford: Oxford University Press).

Lee K. ed. (2002), *Health Impacts of Globalization: Towards Global Governance* (Basingstoke: Palgrave Macmillan).

McMichael A. J. (1993), *Planetary Overload, Global Environmental Change and the Health of the Human Species* (Cambridge: Cambridge University Press).

Reinicke W. (1997), 'Global Public Policy', *Foreign Affairs,* 76(6): 127–38.

Notes

1 An Introduction to Global Health

1 The Gaia Hypothesis was put forth by James Lovelock (1979) who proposes that the Earth and all life on it is an interdependent and self-regulating system that maintains optimal conditions for life.

2 The term Washington Consensus originates from the economist John Williamson (1990) who summarizes his perception of a consensus that emerged by the late 1980s among key political institutions based in Washington (US Congress, Administration, IMF, World Bank, think tanks). He lists ten policy instruments for countries willing to reform their economies, and these ideas have had a major influence on countries around the world. For an analysis of the ideas behind the Washington Consensus, how they have changed over time, and efforts to go beyond the consensus see Naim (1999).

3 The per capita daily supply of calories rose from less than 2500 to 2750 between 1990–97 (UNDP 1999).

4 The Gini coefficient is a commonly used measure of inequality with 0 signifying perfect equality and 100 meaning one person holds all the income.

5 The term *high politics* is used in foreign policy analysis as a collective expression for certain issue areas seen to be of crucial importance to national interests. High politics involves maintenance of core values, including national self-preservation, and the long-term objectives of the state. In situations of conflict, it is implied that foreign policy issues take precedence over domestic or *low politics* issues. Social welfare issues, including health, have traditionally been cast as domestic concerns and thus of lower priority in situations where national interests are at risk (Evans and Newnham 1992: 127).

6 This has largely been pursued through the adoption and enforcement of stronger and more uniform intellectual property laws within the GATT, WTO and World Intellectual Property Organisation (WIPO).

7 For example 95 per cent of all the scientists and technologists who ever lived are currently living. As quoted by P. Kennedy, (1998), 'On thinking and writing about the future', Presentation to ACUNS/ASIL Summer Workshop on Globalization and Global Governance, Yale University, New Haven, August.

8 This is a term used by Antonio Gramsci to describe an earlier form of globalization during the Enlightenment. Q. Hoare, ed. (1977), *Antonio Gramsci, Selections from the Political Writings, 1910–20* (New York: International Publishers), p. 12. See also A. Sassoon, (1997), *Gramsci's Politics, Second Edition* (Minneapolis: University of Minnesota).

9 The General Agreement on Trade in Services (GATS) signed at the Uruguay Round excludes health services. However, regional negotiations and future world trade negotiations seek to include health and other public services

within existing trade law. See A. Pollock and D. Price, (2000) for a discussion.

2   Globalization and Health; A Historical Perspective

1 Beriberi is a disease that causes inflammation of the nerves because of a dietary lack of vitamin B1 (thiamine). It results in fever, paralysis, palpitations and occasionally heart failure. The disease mainly occurs in countries where the staple diet is polished rice. The search for preservation methods during the nineteenth century led to new methods of polishing rice involving the removal of the outer husk. Similar techniques were developed for milling flour to remove the wheat germ and bran. The result is a reduction in nutritional value and an increased risk of vitamin deficiency.
2 The estimated life expectancy among the upper middle class in Manchester was 38 years, and 17 years among the labouring class (Doyal 1979: 50–51).
3 Early examples of international health cooperation include the Superior Council of Health founded in 1838 in Constantinople (Istanbul) with Ottoman and European representation, and the International Board of Health in Tangier, Algeria created in 1840.
4 For a detailed history of WHO prior to the 1970s see WHO (1958), *The First Ten Years of the World Health Organization* (Geneva: WHO) and N. Goodman, (1971), *International Health Organizations and Their Work* (London: Livingstone Churchill).
5 Other health-related UN organizations formed during the postwar period were the UN International Children's Emergency Fund (UNICEF), later renamed the UN Children's Fund, UN Relief and Rehabilitation Administration (UNRRA) and UN High Commissioner for Refugees (UNHCR).

3   The Spatial Dimension of Global Health

1 The term documented migrant is used here to describe people who cross state boundaries in a legally recognized manner subject to the border controls of the country in question. Such travellers are captured on official data on population mobility. It excludes undocumented migrants namely those who travel illicitly and thus seek to circumvent national borders.
2 This term is used to describe the large-scale raising of a relatively small range of species and/or varieties of a crop (e.g. monocropping) in contrast with the practice of encouraging a wide range of species and/or varieties to improve biodiversity.
3 In comparison, HIV/AIDS kills three million people annually, tuberculosis two million and malaria one million (WHO 1996b).

4   The Temporal Dimension of Global Health

1 According to Moore's Law, coined by Gordon Moore, the founder of the silicon chip producer Intel, the processing power of computer chips doubles every eighteen months.

2 Levine (1997) measures pace of life by the speed with which pedestrians in city centres walk 60 feet (walking speed), how quickly postal clerks complete a standard request to purchase a stamp (working speed), and the accuracy of public clocks.

3 Overweight in adults is defined as a body mass index of ≥ 25 and obesity in adults is defined as body mass index ≥ 30. BMI is calculated by weight in kilograms divided by the square of the height in metres (WHO 1997a).

4 It is estimated that the number of drivers on American roads continues to increase, with 91 per cent of people driving to work. In one-third of the largest US cities, commuters spend over 40 hours per year in traffic jams (www.statefarm.com/consumer/crash3.htm).

5 The GM maize is designed to produce a bacterial insecticide, *Bacillus thuringiensis* (Bt), an insecticide commonly used by organic farmers to control the European corn borer.

6 This is measured by a country's 'ecological footprint' defined as the amount of biologically productive land area available per capita. Countries can have an ecological deficit or surplus depending on their available ecological capacity minus their ecological footprint (hectares per capita) (Wackernagel and Callejas 1995).

5   The Cognitive Dimension of Global Health

1 The ten policy recommendations of the Washington Consensus described by Williamson (1990) are: (a) fiscal discipline; (b) redirection of public expenditure; (c) tax reform; (d) financial liberalization; (e) single, competitive exchange rate; (f) trade liberalization; (g) elimination of barriers to foreign direct investment; (h) privatization of state-owned enterprises; (i) deregulation of market entry and competition; and (j) assurance of secure property rights. For a discussion of the origins of, and follow-up to, these ideas see M. Naim (1999), 'Fads and Fashions in Economic Reforms: Washington Consensus or Washington Confusion?' *Foreign Policy Magazine*, 26 October.

2 For comparative analysis of health sector reforms across countries see C. Altenstetter and J. Warner Björkman eds. (1997), *Health Policy Reform, National Variations and Globalization* (Basingstoke: Macmillan – now Palgrave Macmillan); A. Coulter and C. Ham eds. (2000), *The Global Challenge of Health Care Rationing* (Milton Keynes: Open University Press); and A. Mills ed. (2000), *Reforming Health Sectors* (London: Kegan Paul, International).

3 *Fortune* magazine estimates that the global water market is worth US$280 billion annually, 40 per cent of the size of the oil industry and one-third larger than pharmaceuticals. It ranks water as the best investment sector of the century. Similarly, the World Bank estimates the current value of the market at more than US$1 trillion (Tremolet 2001).

4 The staff director of the WDR (2000), Ravi Kanbur, resigned from his role at the World Bank in June 2000 in protest over the report's draft content including its failure to give greater emphasis to income redistribution ('Author of key World Bank report resigns', *Financial Times*, 15 June 2000).

5 GOBI-FFF stands for growth monitoring, oral rehydration, breastfeeding, immunization, female education, family spacing and food supplements.

6 The 10/90 gap describes the situation where less than 10 per cent of global spending on health research is devoted to diseases or conditions that account for 90 per cent of the global burden of disease.

7 Minor financial ties include such interests as ownership of publicly traded mutual funds and honorariums for lectures. The journal continues to prohibit publications from individuals with significant financial interest such as holding company stock or having received more than US$10,000 in the two years before publication.

8 In this chapter, the term advertising is used broadly to include marketing, advertising and sponsorship activities.

9 For a detailed discussion of TTCs and the cognitive dimension of globalization, see Collin (2002).

10 A campaign led by Professor Stanton Glantz of the University of California, San Francisco, a long-time campaigner against TTCs, against the depiction of smoking in film elicited an advertisement in the entertainment publication *Variety* that the campaign was an example of 'tobacco fascism'.

11 It is estimated that each day's delay in getting a major drug to market costs US$1.3 million in unrealized sales (Flaherty et al. 2000).

6 Conclusion: An Agenda for Global Health

1 The international sale of pharmaceuticals through the internet is a rapidly growing business and a direct challenge for national authorities to regulate. Among the *InternetWeek* top 100 companies involved in electronic or e-commerce is American Home Products (AHP) with a projected internet-based revenue growth in 2001 of more than 40 per cent (Violino 2001).

2 Others prefer the broader concept of 'telehealth' which goes beyond the clinical to refer to the use of ICTs to promote, improve and maintain health.

3 A major multidisciplinary study by the Rockefeller Foundation and Swedish International Development Cooperation Agency (SIDA) on *Challenging Inequities in Health* (2001) gives welcome and systematic attention to conceptualizing and empirically measuring health inequities within and across countries. However, the focus of the methodology remains the territorial state.

4 The term natural capital refers to the complete stock of the earth's natural assets such as arable soil, fresh water, animal and plant species and clean air. It also includes the life support systems which are maintained by the planet itself, notably the water cycle, carbon cycle, protective capacity of the ozone layer, and waste-absorbing abilities of land, air and water (Ellwood 2000).

5 The concept of social capital broadly concerns various forms, and the degree, of links that bind together members of a society. These links can take the form of civil society groups, shared cultural and ethnic identities, religious organizations, trade unions, and sporting teams, as well as informal social networks (Harper 2001).

6 Global trade in capital totals US$2 trillion per day. It is estimated that 1–2 per cent is accounted for by foreign exchange transactions related to trade and foreign direct investment. The remainder is for speculation or

short-term investments that can move quickly back out of the country. The rapid increase in global trading has been enabled by financial deregulation and liberalization, technological developments enabling almost instantaneous transactions, and global interconnectedness of capital markets (Khor 1999).

7 One hundred and forty-eight countries attended the first session of the INB in October 2000 (WHO 2000a).

8 For a more detailed discussion of the FCTC and global governance, on which this section is based, see J. Collin, K. Lee and K. Bissell (2002), 'The Framework Convention on Tobacco Control: the politics of global health governance', *Third World Quarterly*, 23(2): 265–82.

9 The Program for Monitoring Emerging Diseases (ProMed) is an initiative of the Federation of American Scientists launched in 1993 for the global monitoring of emerging diseases. The initiative has led to the creation of a global electronic reporting system (ProMED-mail), a public electronic network for reporting outbreaks of infectious human, animal and plant diseases (now operated by the International Society for Infectious Diseases) and Animal Health/Emerging Animal Disease (AHEAD) on the surveillance of infectious animal and zoonotic diseases.

References

Abrams F. (2000), 'Tobacco firm may face inquiry over "smuggling"', *The Guardian*, 17 February.

Allison D., Fontaine K., Manson J., Stevens J., and Van Ittalie T. (1999), 'Annual deaths attributable to obesity in the United States', *Journal of the American Medical Association*, 282: 1530–8.

Altenstetter C. and Björkman J. (1997), 'Globalized concepts and localized practices: convergence and divergence in national health policy reforms' in *Health Policy Reform, National Variations and Globalization* (Basingstoke: Macmillan – now Palgrave Macmillan): 1–16.

Altman D. (1996), 'Rupture or Continuity? The Internationalization of Gay Identities,' *Social Text*, 14(3): 78–94.

Amin S. (1997), *Capitalism in the Age of Globalization* (London: Zed Books).

Anderson S. and Cavanagh J. (2000), 'Top 200, the Rise of Corporate Global Power', Institute for Policy Studies, Washington DC.

Anderson R. and May R. (1991), *Infectious Diseases of Humans, Dynamics and Control* (Oxford: Oxford University Press).

Annan K. (2000), 'Secretary General Statement to General Assembly', 'We the Peoples', The Role of the United Nations in the 21st Century, The Millennium Assembly and the Millennium Summit (New York: United Nations)

Appleby J. (1997), 'Great Britons', *Health Service Journal*, 18 July: 24–25.

Archibald G. (2002), 'Child sex book given out at U.N. summit', *Washington Times*, 10 May.

Arendt A., Echelmeyer K., Harrison W., Lingle C. and Valentine V. (2002), 'Rapid Wastage of Alaska Glaciers and Their Contribution to Rising Sea Level', *Science*, 297, 19 July: 382–6.

Armstrong T. (1995), *The Myth of the A.D.D. Child* (New York: Dutton).

Aron J. L. and Patz J. A., eds. *Ecosystem Change and Public Health, A Global Perspective* (Baltimore: Johns Hopkins University Press).

Astill J. (2001), 'The disappearing apes of Africa', *The Guardian*, 4 July: 2–4 (G2).

'Author of key World Bank report resigns,' *Financial Times*, 15 June 2000.

Barks-Ruggles E. (2001), 'The Globalization of Disease, when Congo sneezes, will California get a cold?' *Brookings Review*, 19(4): 30–3.

Barthold S. (1996), 'Globalization of Lyme borreliosis', *Lancet*, 14 December: 1603–4.

Bartrip P. (1998), 'Too little, too late? The Home Office and the Asbestos Industry Regulations, 1931', *Medical History*, 42: 421–38.

BAT (2001a), *Annual Review and Summary of Financial Statements 2000* (London: BAT Industries, 2001).

BAT (2001b), 'Our history', <www.bat.co.uk> (accessed 31 July 2001).

Beaglehole R. and Bonita R. (1997), *Public Health at the Crossroads: Achievements and prospects* (Cambridge: Cambridge University Press).

Benatar S. (2001), 'Commentary: Justice and Medical Research: A Global Perspective', *Bioethics*, 15(4): 333–40.

Benyon J. and Dunkerley D., eds (2000), *Globalization: The Reader* (London: Athlone Press).

Berer M. (1997), 'Why Reproductive Health and Rights: Because I am a Woman', *Reproductive Health Matters*, 10, November: 16–20.

Beringer J. (1999), 'Keeping watch over genetically modified crops and food', *The Lancet*, 353 (9153), 20 February: 605–6.

Berlan J. P. and Lewontin R. (1999), 'It's business as usual', *The Guardian*, 22 February.

Berlinguer G. (1992), 'The Interchange of Disease and Health between the Old and New Worlds', *American Journal of Public Health*, October, 82(10): 1407–13.

Berridge V. (1999), *Health and Society in Britain since 1939* (Cambridge: Cambridge University Press).

Bettcher D. and Yach D. (1998), 'The Globalization of Public Health Ethics?' *Millennium*, 27(3): 1–28.

Bettcher D., Subramanian C., Guindon E., Perucic A. M., Soll L., Grabham G., Joossens L. and Taylor A. (2001), 'Confronting the Tobacco Epidemic in an Era of Trade Liberalization', Commission on Macroeconomics and Health, Working Paper Series No. WG4:8, Geneva.

Beyer P. (1994), *Religion and Globalization* (London: Sage).

Bigwood J. (2001), 'Toxic Drift – Monsanto and the Drug War in Colombia', *Corporate Watch*, 21 July. <www.purefood.org/monsanto/toxicdrift.cfm> (accessed 27/07.01)

Bioembergen N. (1997), 'A discussion of human population growth', *Carrying Capacity Network Focus*, 7(1).

Birn A. E. and Solarzano A. (1999), 'Public health policy paradoxes: science and politics in the Rockefeller Foundation's hookworm campaign in Mexico in the 1920s', *Social Science and Medicine*, 49(9): 1197–213.

Bishop D., Entwistle P., Cameron I., Allen C., Possee R. (1988), 'Genetically engineered baculovirus insecticides', *Aspects of Applied Biology*, 17: 385–95.

Blair T. (2000), 'Values and the Power of Community', Speech to the Global Ethics Foundation, Tübigen University, Germany, 30 June.

Bloom D. and Canning D. (2000), 'The Health and Wealth of Nations', *Science*, 287; 18 February: 119–20.

Bond P. (1999), 'Globalization, Pharmaceutical Pricing, and South African Health Policy: 'Managing Confrontation with U.S. Firms and Politicians', *International Journal of Health Services*, 29(4): 765–92.

Bonn D. and Bonn J. (2000), 'Work-related stress: can it be a thing of the past?' *The Lancet*, 355, 8 January: 124.

Borger J. (2001), 'Dying for drugs, volunteers or victims? Concern grows over control of drug trials', *The Guardian*, 14 February: 4.

Boseley S. (2001a), 'Legal roadshow rolls on to Brazil', *The Guardian*, 20 April: 13

Boseley S. (2001b), 'Upwardly mobile', *The Guardian*, 1 March: G2.

Brand H., Camaroni I., Gill N., MacLehose L., McKee M., Reintjes R., Schaefer O. and Weinberg J. (2000), *An evaluation of the arrangements for managing an epidemiological emergency involving more than one EU member state* (Bielefeld, Germany: Institute of Public Health).

Branigan T. (2001), 'In the eye of the beholder, Black and Asian women are spending thousands on plastic surgery – to look more Caucasian', *The Guardian*, 15 October: 10.

Bretton Woods Project (2001), 'Global health fund debated', <www.bretton-woodsproject.org/topic/social/s23healthfund.html>

Broughton M. (2001), Speech at the British American Tobacco Annual General Meeting, London, 2 May.

Brown A. (2000), 'Demand for Organic Food Overwhelms UK Farmers', *PA News*, 25 October. <www.purefood.org/Organic/ukorganic/cfm>

Brown D. (2002), 'Human Clone's Birth Predicted, Delivery Outside U.S. May Come by 2003, Researcher Says', *Washington Post*, 16 May: A08.

Brown P. (2002a), 'Mexico's vital gene reservoir polluted by modified maize', *The Guardian*, 19 April: 19.

Brown P. (2002b), 'Why the Mighty Oak Faces Sudden Death', *The Guardian*, 4 May.

Brown P. (2002c), 'Who is to blame? global warming, pulling the plug: why saving energy is the world's most burning issue', Special supplement, *The Guardian*, January 2002.

Brundtland G. H. (2000a), 'Health and Population', BBC Reith Lecture, London.<http://news.bbc.co.uk/hi/english/static/events/reith_2000/lecture 4.stm>

Brundtland G. H. (2000b), WHO Director-General's Response to the Tobacco Hearings, Statement WHO/6, 13 October, <http://www.who.int/genevahearings/hearingsdocs/dghearingsen.rtf> (accessed: 28 October 2001).

Brundtland G. H. (2001a), 'Coping with Stress and Depression in Europe, "Mental Health: A Priority for World Action,"' Speech, Brussels, 25 October. <www.who.int/director-general>

Brundtland G. H. (2001b), 'Globalization as a Force for Better Health', Lecture presented at the Centre for the Study of Global Governance, London School of Economics, London, 16 March.

Bruno K. and Karliner J. (2000), 'Tangled up in Blue, Corporate Partnerships in the UN', Transnational Resource and Action Centre, September. <www.corp watch.org>

Buse K. and Walt G. (2000), 'Global public–private partnerships: part I – a new development in health?' 78(4): 549–61.

Butler P., Hall T., Hanna A., Mendoca L., Auguste B., Manyika J. and Sahay A. (1997), 'A Revolution in Interaction', *McKinsey Quarterly*, 1.

Cairncross F. (1997), *The Death of Distance* (Cambridge Mass.: Harvard Business School Press).

Cann R. (2001), 'Genetic Clues to Dispersal in Human Populations: Retracing the Past from the Present', *Science*, 2 March, 291: 1742–8.

Carlson E., Jacobvitz D. and Sroufe L. A. (1995), 'A Developmental Investigation of Inattentiveness and Hyperactivity', *Child Development*, 66: 37–54.

Carmichael A. (1997), 'Bubonic plague: The Black Death' in Kiple K. ed. *Plague, Pox & Pestilence, Disease in History* (London: Weidenfeld & Nicolson).

Carroll, L. (1865), *Alice's Adventures in Wonderland* (London: Macmillan).

Carslaw N. (2001), '"Record demand" for organic food', BBC News, 26 March. <http://news.bbc.co.uk>

Casidio Tarabusi C. and Vickery G. (1998), 'Globalization in the Pharmaceutical Industry, Part I', *International Journal of Health Services*, 28(1): 67–105.

Castleman B. (1995), 'The Migration of Industrial Hazards', *International Journal of Occupational and Environmental Health*, 1(2): 85–96.

Castleman B. (1999), 'Global Corporate Policies and International "Double Standards" in Occupational and Environmental Health', *International Journal of Occupational and Environmental Health*, 5(1): 61–4.

Castleman B. and Lemen R. (1998), 'The Manipulation of International Scientific Organizations,' *International Journal of Occupational and Environmental Health*, 4(1): 53–5.

Castleman B. and Navarro V. (1987), 'International Mobility of Hazardous Products, Industries, and Wastes', *Annual Review of Public Health*, 8: 1–19.

CDC (2002), *Prevalence of Attention Deficit Disorder and Learning Disability* (Atlanta: US Centers for Disease Control and Prevention).

Cernea M. ed. (1999); *The Economics of Involuntary Resettlement: Questions and Answers* (Washington DC: World Bank).

Chaloupka F. and Laixuthai A. (1996), US Trade Policy and Cigarette Smoking in Asia, Working Paper No. 5543, Cambridge, Mass: National Bureau of Economic Research.

Chan R. (2001), 'The Sustainability of the Asian Welfare System after the Financial Crisis: Reflections on the Case of Hong Kong,' *SEARC Working Paper Series No. 7*, City University of Hong Kong, May.

Chang R. and Majnoni G. (2000), 'International Contagion, Implications for Policy,' Policy Research Working Paper, No. 2306, World Bank, Washington DC, March.

Chantornvong S. and McCargo D. (2001), 'Political economy of tobacco control in Thailand,' *Tobacco Control*, 10: 48–54.

Chetley A. (1995), 'Pill Pushers, Drug Dealers', *New Internationalist*, October, 272: 22–3.

Chisholm N. (2002), 'Africans destroy skin as they seek to lighten complexion', *Village Voice* (New York), reprinted in *The Guardian*, 29 January.

Clark A. (2001), 'Glaxo relents on Aids drugs', *The Guardian*, 22 April: 25.

Cliff A. and Haggett P. (1989), 'Spatial aspects of epidemic control', *Progress in Human Geography*, 13(3): 315–47.

Cohen J. (1996), 'Maximum occupancy', *American Demographics*, 18(2): 50–1.

Cohen M. (1989), *Health and the Rise of Civilization* (New Haven: Yale University Press).

Coiera E. (1996), 'The Internet's challenge to health care provision,' BMJ, 312, 6 January: 3–4.

Collin J. (2002), 'Think global, smoke local: Transnational tobacco companies and cognitive globalization', in Lee K. ed. (2002), *Health Impacts of Globalization: Towards Global Governance* (London: Palgrave Macmillan): 61–85.

Collin, J. and Lee, K. (2003) *Globalisation and Transborder Health Risk in the UK: Case Studies in Tobacco Control and Population Mobility* (London: Nuffield Trust).

Collin J., Lee K. and Bissell K. (2002), 'The Framework Convention on Tobacco Control: the politics of global health governance', *Third World Quarterly*, 23(2): 265–82.

Colwell R. (1996), 'Global climate and infectious disease: the cholera paradigm', *Science*, 274: 2025–31.

Commission on Global Governance (1995), *Our Global Neighbourhood, The Report of the Commission on Global Governance* (London: Oxford University Press).

Connor S. (1988), 'Genes on the loose', *New Scientist*, 26 May: 65–8.

Consumers International (1997), 'Consumer Charter for Global Business', London, October. <www.consumersinternational.org/campaigns/trade/charter_en.html>

Consumers International (2001), 'Corporate Citizenship in the Global Market, Accountability and the Consumer Perspective', <www.consumersinternational.org> (accessed 5 May 2002).

Cooper C. (2001), '"I can't cope anymore"', *The Guardian*, 5 November.

Copeland R. (2002), 'An ethical dimension', *AUTLook*, 220, January: 4.

Cornea G. A. (2001), 'Globalization and Health: results and options', *Bulletin of the World Health Organization*, 79(9): 834–41

Corrigan T. (1999), 'Cross-border M&A deals at record levels', *Financial Times*, 5 April: 16.

Coulter A. and Ham C., eds (2000), *The Global Challenge of Health Care Rationing* (Milton Keynes: Open University Press).

Cox H. (2000), *The Global Cigarette, Origins and Evolution of British American Tobacco* (Oxford: Oxford University Press).

Cox R. W. (1987), *Production, Power and World Order, Social Forces in the Making of History* (New York: Columbia University Press).

Cox R. W. (1995), 'Critical Political Economy' in Hettne B. ed. *International Political Economy, Understanding Global Disorder* (London: Zed Books): 31–45.

Coyle D. (2001), 'Analysis: Globalising Doom', Transcript of BBC Radio 4 Production, London 15 November. <www.bbc.co.uk> (accessed 15 January 2002).

Craft N. (1994), 'Food irradiation is safe, says WHO', *British Medical Journal*, 309, 29 October: 1110.

Crosby A. W. (1972), *The Columbian Exchange, Biological and Cultural Consequences of 1492* (Westport, Conn.: Greenwood Press).

Crosby A. W. (1986), *Ecological Imperialism, The Biological Expansion of Europe, 900–1900* (London: Canto).

Cross-National Collaborative Group (1992), 'The changing rate of major depression: cross-national comparisons', *Journal of the American Medical Association*, 268(21), 2 December: 3098–105.

de Cock K., Lucas S., Mabey D. and Parry E. (1995), 'Tropical medicine for the 21st century', *British Medical Journal*, 30 September, 311: 860–2.

DeGrandpre R. (1999), *Ritalin Nation, Rapid-Fire Culture and the Transformation of Human Consciousness* (New York: W.W. Norton).

De Zulueta J. (1987), 'Changes in the Geographical Distribution of Malaria throughout History', *Parassitologia*, 29: 193–205.

De Zulueta J. (1994), 'Malaria and Ecosystems: From Prehistory to Posteradication', *Parissitologia*, 36: 7–15.

Deacon B., Hulse M. and Stubbs P. (1997), *Global Social Policy, International Organizations and the Future of Welfare* (London: Sage).

Desowitz R. S. (1997), *Who Gave Pinta to the Santa Maria? Tracking the Devastating Spread of Lethal Tropical Diseases into America* (New York: Harcourt Brace).

Devlin, N., Maynard, A. and Mays, N. (2001). 'New Zealand's new health sector reforms: back to the future?' *British Medical Journal* 322: 1171–4.

Dicken P. (1998), *Global Shift: Transforming the World Economy*, 3rd edition (London: Sage).

Dietz W. (1998), 'Prevalence of obesity in children' in Bray G., Bouchard C. and James W. eds, *Handbook of Obesity* (New York: Marcel Dekker): 93–102.

Dikhanov Y. and Ward M. (2001), 'Measuring the distribution of global income', Background Paper for Poverty Net, World Bank, Washington DC.

Dobyns H. (1966), 'Estimating Aboriginal American Population,' *Current Anthropology*, 7: 395–449.

Dodgson R., Lee K. and Drager N. (2002), 'Global health governance: A conceptual review', *Briefing Paper No. 1*, WHO Department of Health and Development, Geneva.

Doll R. and Hill A. (1950), 'Smoking and carcinoma of the lung: preliminary report,' *British Medical Journal*, 143: 329–36.

Dollar D. and Kraay A. (2000), 'Growth is Good for the Poor', *Discussion Paper*, Development Research Group, World Bank, Washington DC, March.

Doyal L. (1979), *The Political Economy of Health* (London: Pluto Press).

Doyal L. (1996), 'The politics of women's health: Setting a global agenda', *International Journal of Health Services*, 26(1): 47–65.

Draganescu N., Iftimovici R., Iacobescu V., Girjabu E., Busila A., Cvasniuc D., Tudor G., Lapusneanu C. and Manastireanu M. (1975), 'Investigations on the presence of antibodies to several flaviviruses in humans and some domestic animals in a biotype with a high frequency of migratory birds', *Virologie*, 26(2): 103–8.

Drazen J. and Curfman G. (2002), 'Financial Associations of Authors', *New England Journal of Medicine*, 346(24), 13 June: 1901–2.

Drewnowski A. and Popkin B. (1997), 'The Nutrition Transition: New Trends in the Global Diet', *Nutrition Review*, 55(2): 31–43.

Dubin M. (1995), 'The League of Nations Health Organisation' in Weindling P. ed. *International Health Organisations and Movements, 1918–1939* (Cambridge: Cambridge University Press): 56–80.

Dunwell J. (1999), 'Transgenic Crops: The Next Generation, or an Example of 2020 Vision', *Annals of Botany*, 84: 269–77.

Dyches H. and Rushing B. (1996), 'International stratification and the health of women: an empirical comparison of alternative models of world-system position', *Social Science and Medicine*, 43(7): 1063–72.

El Wardani, N. (2003), Did procedural justice exist in policy process for health sector reform in Egypt? Unpublished paper, London School of Hygiene and Tropical Medicine.

Ellwood W. (2000), 'Let's stop ransacking the Earth and start searching for sustainability', *New Internationalist*, November, 329.

Ellwood W. (2001), *The No-Nonsense Guide to Globalization* (London: Verso).

Eltis D., Behrendt S., Richardson D. and Klein H. (1999), *The Transatlantic Slave Trade: A Database on CD-ROM* (Cambridge: Cambridge University Press).

Ende M. (1984), *Momo* (Harmondsworth: Penguin).

Engel C. (2001a), 'Playing the wild card,' *Financial Times*, 16 June.

Engel, C. (2001b), *Wild Health* (London: Weidenfeld and Nicolson).

EURODIAB ACE Study Group (2000), 'Variation and trends in incidence of childhood diabetes in Europe', *The Lancet*, 355: 873–6.

Evans G. and Newnham J. (1992), *The Dictionary of World Politics* (London: Harvester Wheatsheaf).

Falk R. (1999), *Predatory Globalization, A Critique* (Cambridge: Polity Press).

Fanning E. A. (1998), 'Globalization of tuberculosis', *Canadian Medical Association Journal*, 158(5): 10 March: 611–12.

Farley J. (1995), 'The International Health Division of the Rockefeller Foundation: the Russell years, 1920–1934' in Weindling P. ed., *International Health Organisations and Movements, 1918–1939* (Cambridge: Cambridge University Press): 203–21.

Farmer P. (2001), *Infections and Inequalities, The Modern Plague* 2nd edition (Berkeley: University of California Press).

Farrelly P. (2001a), 'Big … and plotting to become bigger still', *The Observer*, 22 April: 3.

Farrelly P. (2001b), 'Glaxo eyes £150bn bid for US rival', *The Observer*, 22 April: B1.

Feachem R. (2001), 'Globalisation is good for your health, mostly', *British Medical Journal*, 323; 1 September 2001: 504–6

Fidler D. (1996), 'Globalization, International Law, and Emerging Infectious Diseases', *Emerging Infectious Diseases*, 2(2): 77–84.

Fidler D. (2001), 'The globalization of public health: the first 100 years of international health diplomacy', *Bulletin of the World Health Organization*, 79(9): 842–9.

Fidler D. (2002), 'Public health and national security in the global age: Infectious diseases, bioterrorism, and Realpolitik', Paper presented at the Centre on Global Change and Health, London School of Hygiene and Tropical Medicine, London, May.

Firn D. (2001), 'Solvay gets approval for new production of flu vaccine', *Financial Times*, 28 June.

Flaherty M., Nelson D. and Stephens J. (2000), 'The Body Hunters, Part 2: Overwhelming the Watchdogs', *Washington Post*, 18 December: A01.

Flavin C. (1996), 'Facing Up to the Risks of Climate Change' in Brown L. ed., *State of the World* (New York: W.W. Norton).

Francey N. and Chapman S. (2000), '"Operation Berkshire": the international tobacco companies' conspiracy', *British Medical Journal*, 5 August, 321; 371–74.

French H. (2000), *Vanishing Borders, Protecting the Planet in the Age of Globalization* (New York: W.W. Norton).

Frenk J. (1994), 'Dimensions of health sector reform', *Health Policy*, 27: 19–34.

Frenk, J. and Sepulveda J. (1997), 'The new world order and international health.' *British Medical Journal* 314(7091): 1404–1407.

Frühbeck G. (2000), 'Childhood obesity: time for action, not complacency,' *British Medical Journal*, 320; 5 February: 328–9.

Gallant R. (1990), *The Peopling of Planet Earth: Human population growth through the ages* (New York: Macmillan).

Gao F., Bailes E., Robertson D., Chen Y., Rodenburg C., Michael S., Cummins L., Arthur L., Peeters M., Shaw G., Sharp P. and Hahn B. (1999), 'Origin of HIV-1 in the chimpanzee Pan troglodytes troglodytes', *Nature*, 397 (6718), 4 February: 385–6.

Garrett L. (1994), *The Coming Plague: Newly Emerging Diseases in a World Out of Balance* (New York: Farrar, Straus & Giroux).

Garrett L. (2000), '"You just signed his death warrant": AIDS Politics and the Journalists' Role', *Columbia Journalism Review*, November/December.

Garrett L. (2001), *Betrayal of Trust, the Collapse of Global Public Health* (Oxford: Oxford University Press).

George S. (1999), 'Neo-liberalism – an introduction', Paper presented at the Conference on Economic Sovereignty in a Globalising World, Bangkok, 24–26 March.

Gernhart G. (1999), 'A Forgotten Enemy: PHS's Fight against the 1918 Influenza Pandemic', *Public Health Reports*, November/December, 114(6): 559–61.

Giddens A. (1990), *The Consequences of Modernity* (Stanford: Stanford University Press).

Giddens A. (1998), *The Third Way, The Renewal of Social Democracy* (Cambridge: Polity Press).

Gill S. (1997), 'Gramsci, modernity and globalization,' Paper presented to the Annual Conference of the British International Studies Association, University of Leeds, December.

Gillam C. (2001), 'Gene Giants Criticized at World Ag Forum', Organic Consumers Association <www.purefood.org/monsanto/toomuchpower.cfm> (accessed 27.07.01).

Gilmore A., McKee M. and Rose R. (2002), 'Determinants of and inequalities in self-perceived health in the Ukraine,' *Social Science and Medicine*.

Gittings J. (2001), 'China's children labour round the clock', *The Guardian*, 26 September: 14.

Gleick J. (1999), *Faster: The acceleration of just about everything* (New York: Little, Brown).

Global Forum for Health Research (2000), *The 10/90 Report on Health Research* (Geneva: WHO).

Global Fund to Fight AIDS, Tuberculosis & Malaria website <www.globalfundatm.org>

Godlee F. (1994), 'WHO in Crisis', *British Medical Journal*, 309, 26 November: 1424–8.

Goldsmith E. (1996), 'Global Trade and the Environment' in Mander J. and Goldsmith E. eds, *The Case Against the Global Economy* (San Francisco: Sierra Club): 78–91.

Goodman N. (1971), *International Health Organizations and Their Work* (London: Livingstone Churchill).

Gottdiener M. (1994), *The Social Production of Urban Space* (Austin: University of Texas Press).

Grein T., Kande-Bure O., Rodier G., Plant A., Bovier P., Ryan M., Ohyama T. and Heymann D. (2000), 'Rumors of Disease in the Global Village: Outbreak Verification,' *Emerging Infectious Diseases*, 6(2): 97–102.

GSK (2001), *Annual Report 2000* (Greenford: GlaxoSmithKline). <www.gsk.com>

Gupte S and Gupta R. (2002), 'India's summer cola wars', *Adage Global*, 28 March. <www.adageglobal.com>

Gwatkin D., Guillot M. and Heuveline P. (1999), 'The burden of disease among the global poor,' *The Lancet*, 354; 14 August: 586–9.

Haas P. (1992), 'Introduction: Epistemic Communities and International Policy Coordination', *International Organization*, 46(1): 1–20.

Haines A. and McMichael A. J. (1997) 'Climate change and health: implication for research, monitoring and policy,' *British Medical Journal*, 315, 4 October: 870–4.

Hallowell E. and Ratey J. (1995), *Driven to Distraction* (New York: Pantheon).

Hammond R. (1998), *Addicted to Profit: Big Tobacco's Expanding Global Reach* (Washington DC: Essential Action).

Hannerz U. (1991), 'Scenarios for peripheral cultures' in King A. ed., *Culture, Globalization and the World System* (New York: State University of New York).

Hardt M. and Negri A. (2000), *Empire* (Cambridge, Mass.: Harvard University Press).

Harper R. (2001), *Social Capital, A Review of the Literature* (London: Office for National Statistics).

Harris P. (2001), *The History of Human Populations, Vol. I: Forms of Growth and Development* (New York: Praeger).

Harvey F. (2000a), 'Information at the bedside: Just what the doctor ordered ... over the internet', *Financial Times*, 28 November.

Harvey F. (2000b), 'The processors at the heart of healthcare', *Financial Times*, 29 November: 20.

Hastings G. and MacFadyen L. (2000), *Keep Smiling: No One's Going to Die. An analysis of internal documents from the tobacco industry's main UK advertising agencies* (London: British Medical Association). <www.ctcr.strath.ac.uk/links.htlm>

Hays J. N. (1998), *The Burdens of Disease, Epidemics and Human Response in Western History* (New Brunswick, N. J.: Rutgers University Press).

Health Canada (1999), 'GPHIN', April. <www.hc-sc.gc.ca/ohih-bsi/nhsi_e.html>

Health Canada (2000), 'What is the population health approach?' <www.hc-sc.gc.ca/hppb/phdd/approach/index.html> (accessed March 2001).

Held D., McGrew A., Goldblatt D. and Perraton J. (1999), *Global Transformations, Politics, Economics and Culture* (Stanford: Stanford University Press).

Henderson M. (2000), 'Threat that never was', *The Times (Science Supplement)*, 14 December: 12–13.

Hirst P. and Thompson G. (1995), 'Globalization and the future of the nation state', *Economy and Society*, 24(3): 408–42.

Hoare Q. ed. (1977), *Antonio Gramsci, Selections from the Political Writings, 1910–20* (New York: International Publishers).

Holden C. (2000), 'Global Survey Examines Impact of Depression', *Science*, 288; 7 April, 39–40.

Horsey K. (2002), 'HFEA makes tissue typing decision', *BioNews*, 1 March.

Hutton W. (2003), *The World We're In* (London: Abacus)

IBFAN (2001), 'Multinational baby food companies Nestlé, Milupa, Abbott-Ross, Mead-Johnson and Wyeth are the worst violators of the International Code of Marketing of Breastmilk Substitutes, says IBFAN', *Press Release*, Geneva, 15 May.

ICAF (1996), *Transportation Industry Study Report 1996* (Washington DC: National Defence University, Industrial College of the Armed Forces).

ICFTU (1998), *Fighting for Workers' Human Rights in the Global Economy* (Brussels: International Confederation of Free Trade Unions).

ICRCRCS (2002), *World Disasters Report 2002* (Geneva: International Federation of Red Cross and Red Crescent Societies).

ILO (2000), 'Globalization may increase number of migrant workers', *Press Release*, Geneva, 2 March.

ILO (2002), *A Future Without Child Labour* (Geneva: International Labour Organization).

Institute of Medicine (1997), *America's Vital Interest in Global Health* (Washington DC: National Academy Press).

Intel (2002), 'Processor Hall of Fame', <www.intel.com> (accessed 14 June 2002).

International Human Genome Sequencing Consortium (2001), 'Initial sequencing and analysis of the human genome', *Nature*, 409, 13 February: 860–921.

International Organization for Migration (1998), 'Trafficking Gets High Level Attention', *Trafficking in Migrants Quarterly Bulletin*, No. 18, June.

Ishiguro F., Takada N., Masuzawa T. and Fukui T. (2000), 'Prevalence of Lyme disease Borrelia spp. in ticks from migratory birds on the Japanese mainland', *Applied Environmental Microbiology*, 66(3): 982–6.

ITU (1998), *World Telecommunication Development Report 1998* (Geneva: International Telecommunication Union).

IWHC (2002), 'International Women's Health Coalition,' <www.iwhc.org>

Jackson J. (1998), 'Cognition and the Global Malaria Eradication Programme', *Parassitologia*, 40: 193–216.

Jameson F. and Miyoshi M. eds. (1998), *The Cultures of Globalization* (Durham, NC: Duke University Press).

Jamison D., Mosley W. H., Measham A. and Bobadilla J. (1993), *Disease Control Priorities in Developing Countries* (Oxford: Oxford University Press/World Bank).

Japan (2001), *White Paper on International Trade* (Tokyo: Ministry of Economy, Trade and Industry). <http://jin.jcic.or.jp/stat/stats/07IND25.html>

Jerardo, A. (2002) 'The Import Share of U.S.-Consumed Food Continues to Rise', Economic Research Service, US Department of Agriculture, July. <www.ers.usda.gov>

Jernigan D. H., Monteiro M., Room R. and Saxena S. (2000), 'Towards a global alcohol policy: alcohol, public health and the role of WHO', *Bulletin of the World Health Organization*, 78(4): 491–9.

Jha P. and Chaloupka F., eds (2000), *Tobacco Control in Developing Countries* (Oxford: Oxford University Press/World Bank).

Jha P. and Mills A. (2002), *Improving Health Outcomes of the Poor*, Report of Working Group 5 of the Commission on Macroeconomics and Health, WHO, Geneva, April.

Johnston D. (2001), 'Harvard scientist warns environmental damage irreversible', *OECD Observer*, 16 May.

Joint M. (1995), *Road Rage*, Report for the Automobile Association Group Public Policy Road Safety Unit, Washington DC.

Jones K. and Moon G. (1987), *Health, Disease and Society: A Critical Medical Geography* (London: Routledge & Kegan Paul).

Jones R. J. B. (1995), *Globalization and Interdependence in the International Political Economy* (London: Pinter).

Jones S. (1997), *In the Blood: God, Genes and Destiny* (London: Flamingo).

Joossens L. (2002), 'Tobacco smuggling', *Tobacco Control Factsheets*, International Union Against Cancer (UICC). <http://factsheets.globalink.org/en/smuggling.html>

Josefson D. (2001), 'Obesity and inactivity fuel global cancer epidemic', *British Medical Journal*, 322; 21 April: 945.

Jowett M. (1999), 'Bucking the trend? Health care expenditures in low-income countries 1990–95', *International Journal of Health Planning and Management*, 14: 269–85.

Ka-Min L. (2000), 'User fees blamed for cholera outbreak in South Africa', Third World Network, <www.twnside.org.sg/title/cholera.htm>

Kaferstein F., Motarjemi Y. and Bettcher D. (1997), 'Foodborne Disease Control – A Transnational Challenge', *Emerging Infectious Diseases*, 3(4): 503–10.

Kalekin-Fishman D. (1996), 'The Impact of Globalization on the Determination and Management of Ethical Choices in the Health Arena', *Social Science and Medicine*, 43(5): 809–22.

Kapitsa S. (1997), 'A model of world population growth as an experiment in systematic research', *Voprosy Statistiki*, 8: 46–57.

Karlen A. (1995), *Man and Microbes, Disease and Plagues in History and Modern Times* (New York: Simon & Schuster).

Kassalow J. (2001), *Why Health Is Important to U.S. Foreign Policy* (New York: Council on Foreign Relations and Milbank Memorial Fund).

Katz R. S. (1974), 'Influenza 1918-1919: A Study in Mortality', *Bulletin of the History of Medicine*, 48(3): 416–23.

Kaul I. (2001), 'Global Public Goods and the Poor', *Development*, 44(1): 77–84.

Kaul I., Grunberg I. and Stern M. eds (1999), *Global Public Goods, International Cooperation in the 21st Century* (Oxford: Oxford University Press).

Kaul M. (1997), 'The New Public Administration: management innovations in government', *Public Administration and Development*, 17: 13–26.

Keith L. and Del Priore G. (2002), 'Uterine transplantation in humans: a new frontier', *International Journal of Gynecology & Obstetrics*, March, 76(3): 243–4.

Kennedy P. (1996), 'Forecast: global gales ahead', *New Statesman & Society*, 31 May: 28–9.

Kennedy P. (1998), 'On thinking and writing about the future', Presentation to ACUNS/ASIL Summer Workshop on Globalization and Global Governance, Yale University, New Haven, August.

Kessler D. (2001), *A Question of Intent, A Great American Battle with a Deadly Industry* (New York: Public Affairs).

Kewley G. (1998), 'Attention deficit hyperactivity disorder is underdiagnosed and undertreated in Britain', *British Medical Journal*, 316, 23 May: 1594–6.

Khor M. (1999), 'The Economic Crisis in East Asia: Causes, Effects, Lessons', *Discussion Paper*, Third World Network, Kuala Lumpur.

Kickbusch I. (1997), 'New players for a new era: responding to the global public health challenge', *Journal of Public Health Medicine*, 19(2): 171–8.

Killalea D., Ward L., Roberts D. et al. (1996), 'International epidemiological and microbiological study of outbreak of *Salmonella agona* infection from a ready to eat savoury snack – I: England and Wales and the United States', *British Medical Journal*, 313, 2 November: 1105–7.

Klein N. (2000), *No Logo* (New York: HarperCollins/Flamingo).

Kneen B. (1999), 'Restructuring food for corporate profit: The corporate genetics of Cargill and Monsanto', *Agriculture and Human Values*, 16(2): 161–7.

Korten D. (2001), *When Corporations Rule the World, 2nd edition* (London: Kumarian Press).

Kowalczyk L. (2001), 'New steps urged on university research bias,' *Boston Globe*, 21 February: A1.

Lang T. (1997), 'The public health impact of the globalisation of food trade' in Shetty P. and McPherson K. eds, *Diet, Nutrition and Chronic Disease: Lessons from Contrasting Worlds* (London: John Wiley): 173–87.

Lang T. (1998), 'The new globalisation, food and health: is public health receiving its due emphasis?' *Journal of Epidemiology and Community Health*, 52: 538–9.

Lang T. (1999), 'Diet, health and globalization: five key questions', *Proceedings of the Nutrition Society*, 58: 335–43.

Lasagna L. (1997), 'In Pursuit of Profitability and Effectiveness in the Global Pharmaceutical Industry: Comments on Professor Walker's Four Challenges', *Indiana Journal of Global Legal Studies*, 5(1): 85–92.

Lawrence F. (2001), 'We are the masters now', *The Guardian*, 10 August: 11.

Leahy J. (2001), 'Bird virus poses threat to a Hong Kong way of life', *Financial Times*, 28 May.

Lee K. (1998), 'Shaping the future of global health cooperation: where can we go from here?' *The Lancet*, 351, 21 March: 899–902.

Lee K. (2000), 'Globalisation and health policy: A conceptual framework and research and policy agenda' in Bambas A. and Drayton H. eds, *Health and Human Development in the New Global Economy* (Washington DC: Pan American Health Organization): 15–41.

Lee K. (2001a), 'A dialogue of the deaf? The health impacts of globalisation', *Journal of Epidemiology and Community Health*, 55(9): 619–21.

Lee (2001b), 'The global dimensions of cholera', *Global Change and Human Health*, 2(1): 2–15.

Lee K. ed. (2002), *Health Impacts of Globalization: Towards global governance* (London: Palgrave Macmillan).

Lee K., Collinson S., Walt G. and Gilson L. (1996), 'Who should be doing what in international health: A confusion of mandates in the United Nations?' *British Medical Journal*, 312, 3 February: 302–7.

Lee K. and Dodgson R. (2000), 'Globalisation and cholera: Implications for global governance', *Global Governance*, 6(2): 213–36.

Lee K. and Goodman H. (2002), 'Global policy networks: The propagation of health care financing reform since the 1980s' in Lee K., Buse K. and Fustukian S. eds, *Health Policy in a Globalising World* (Cambridge: Cambridge University Press): 97–119.

Lee K. and Patel P. (2002), 'Far from the Maddening Cows: The Global Dimensions of BSE and vCJD' in Lee K. ed., *Health Impacts of Globalization: Towards Global Governance* (Basingstoke: Palgrave Macmillan): 47–60.

Levine R. (1997), *A Geography of Time* (New York: Basic Books).

Link E. and Rossel S. (2001), 'Global tobacco: Where cigarette manufacturers roam', *Tobacco Journal International*, 6 (November/December): 17–20.

Lister G. (2000), 'Programme report and action plan' in Parsons L. and Lister G. eds, *Global Health, A Local Issue* (London: Nuffield Trust): 171–94.

Loewenberg S (2000) 'Tobacco Lights Into WHO Industry Pushes to Influence October Treaty Debate Over Global Curbs on Cigarettes', *Legal Times*, 11 September, <http://lists.essential.org/pipermail/intl-tobacco/2000q3/000276.html> (accessed 28 October 2001).

Loewenson R. (2000), 'Social development and social services under globalisation in Zimbabwe', Paper prepared for the 1999 Zimbabwe Human Development Report, Harare, February.

Longworth R. (1999), 'Activists on Internet Reshaping Rules for Global Economy', *Chicago Tribune*, 5 July.

Losey J., Rayor L. and Carter M. (1999), 'Transgenic crop harms monarch larvae', *Nature*, 399, 20 May: 214

Love J. (1995), *McDonald's Behind the Arches, A History of McDonalds* (New York: Bantam Books).

Lovelock J. (1979), *Gaia* (Oxford: Oxford University Press).

Lucas A., Mogedal S., Walt G., Hodne Steen S., Kruse S. E., Lee K. and Hawken L. (1997), *Cooperation for Health Development: The World Health Organisation's Support to Programmes at the Country Level* (London: Governments of Australia, Canada, Italy, Norway, Sweden and the United Kingdom).

MacAskill E. (1999), 'Tories attack old ally in onslaught on tobacco firm', *The Guardian*, 20 July.

MacKay H. (2000), 'The globalization of culture?' in Held D. ed., *A globalizing world? Culture, economics, politics* (London: Routledge and Open University Press): 47–84.

MacPherson D. (2001), 'Human Health, Demography and Population Mobility', *Migration and Health* (International Organization for Migration), No. 1.

Madison G. G. (1998), *Globalization: Challenges and Opportunities*, GHC Working Paper 98/1.

Maguire K. and Borger J. (2002), 'Scruton in media plot to push the sale of cigarettes', *The Guardian*, 24 January.

Mahathir Bin Mohamed (2002), 'Our experience can help shape a globalization that benefits all', Keynote address to 35th General Meeting of the Pacific Basin Economy Council (PBEC), Beijing, 6 May.

Marmor T. (1994), *Understanding Health Care Reform* (New Haven, Conn.: Yale University Press).

Martens P., Kovats S., Nijhof S., de Vries P., Livermore M., Bradley D., Cox J. and McMichael A. J. (1999), 'Climate change and future populations at risk of malaria', *Global Environmental Change*, 9: S89–107.

May R. (2000), 'The Human Genome Project', Wellcome Trust Sanger Institute, <www.sanger.ac.uk/HGP/draft2000/commentary.html>

McGinn A. P. (1997), 'The Nicotine Cartel', *WorldWatch*, 10(4): 18–27.

McGraw P. (2001), *Life Strategies*, 2nd Edition (New York: Vermillion).

McGreal C. (2001), 'ANC urged to deliver AIDS drugs', *The Guardian*, 20 April: 13.

McKeigue P. and Sevak L. (1994), *Coronary Heart Disease in South Asian Communities, A Manual for Health Promotion* (London: Health Education Authority).

McKie R. (2001), 'Farm virus "came from Africa in a dust storm",' *The Observer*, 9 September: 7.

McKinlay J. and Marceau L. (2002), 'The end of the golden age of doctoring,' *International Journal of Health Services*, 32(2): 379–416.

McMichael A. J. (1993), *Planetary Overload: Global Environmental Change and the Health of the Human Species* (Cambridge: Cambridge University Press).

McMichael A. J. (2000), 'The urban environment and health in a world of increasing globalization: issues for developing countries,' *Bulletin of the World Health Organization*, 78(9): 1117–6.

McMichael A. J. (2001), *Human Frontiers, Environments and Disease* (Cambridge: Cambridge University Press).

McMichael A. J. and Haines A. (1997), 'Global climate change: The potential effects on health,' *British Medical Journal*, 315: 805–9.

McMichael A. J., Bolin B., Constanza R., Daily G., Folke C., Lindahl-Kiessling K., Lindgren E. and Niklasson B., (1999) 'Globalization and the Sustainability of Human Health, an ecological perspective', BioScience, 49(3): 205–10.

McMichael P. (1998), 'Global Food Politics', *Monthly Review*, 50(3): 97–111.

McNeil D. (2002), 'Generic AIDS drugs on UN list', *New York Times*, 21 March.

McNeill W. (1976), *Plagues and People* (New York: Anchor Press/Doubleday).

Meek J. (2001), 'Scientists plan to wipe out malaria with GM mosquitoes', *The Guardian*, 3 September: 3.

Michaud C. and Murray C. (1996), 'Resources for health research and development in 1992: a global overview' in Ad Hoc Committee on Health Research Relating to Future Intervention Options, *Investing in Health Research and Development* (Geneva: WHO).

Milanovic B. (2000), *Income, Inequality and Poverty during the Transition from Planned to Market Economy* (Washington DC: World Bank).

Milanovic B. (2002), 'True world income distribution, 1988 and 1993: First calculation based on household surveys alone', *Economic Journal*, 112, January: 51–92.

Mills A. ed. (2000), *Reforming Health Sectors* (London: Kegan Paul).

Miyamoto K., Sato Y., Okada K., Fukunaga M. and Sato F. (1997), 'Competence of a migratory bird, red-bellied thrush (Turdus chrysolaus), as an avian reservoir for the Lyme disease spirochetes in Japan,' *Acta Tropica*, 65(1): 43–51.

Mizell L. (1996), *Aggressive Driving*, A Report for the AAA Foundation for Traffic Safety, Washington DC.

Mokdad A., Ford E., Bowman B. et al. (2000a), 'Diabetes trends in the United States, 1990–1998,' *Diabetes Care*, 23: 1278–83.

Mokdad A., Serdula M., Dietz W., Bowman B., Marks J. and Koplan J. (2000b), 'The Continuing Epidemic of Obesity in the United States,' *Journal of the American Medical Association*, 284(13); 4 October: 1650–1.

Mokdad A., Bowman B., Ford E., Vinicor F., Marks J. and Koplan J. (2001), 'The Continuing Epidemics of Obesity and Diabetes in the United States', *Journal of the American Medical Association*, 286(10); 12 September: 1195–200.

Monsanto Company (2000a), *2000 Annual Report* (St. Louis: Monsanto Company).

Monsanto Company (2000b), 'Company Timeline/History', St. Louis, <www.monsanto.com/monsanto/about_us/company_timeline/default.htm> (accessed 27 July 2001).

Mooney P. (1999), *The ETC Century, Erosion, Technological Transformation and Corporate Concentration in the 21st Century* (Uppsala: Dag Hammarskjold Foundation/Rural Advancement Foundation International).

Moran M. and Wood B. (1996), 'The Globalization of Health Care Policy?' in Gummett P. ed., *Globalization and Public Policy* (London: Edward Elgar) 125–42.

Moses H. and Martin J. (2001), 'Academic relationships with Industry, A New Model for Biomedical Research', *Journal of the American Medical Association*, 285(7), 21 February: 933–5.

Moyer D. (2000), *The Tobacco Reference Guide* (UICC GLOBALink). <www.globalink.org/tobacco/trg/>

Murphy C. (2000), 'Political consequences of the new inequality', Presidential address to the Annual Conference of the International Studies Association, New Orleans, February.

Murray C. and Lopez A. eds (1996), *The Global Burden of Disease* (Cambridge, Mass.: Harvard University Press/WHO/World Bank).

Murray C., Michaud C., McKenna M. and Marks J. (1994), *US patterns of mortality by country and race: 1965–1994* (Cambridge, Mass.: National Center for

Chronic Disease Prevention and Health Promotion and Harvard Center for Population and Development Studies).

Musto D. (1991), 'Opium, Cocaine and Marijuana in American History', *Scientific American*, July: 20–7.

Naim M. (1999), 'Fads and Fashions in Economic Reforms: Washington Consensus or Washington Confusion?' *Foreign Policy Magazine*, 26 October.

Natsios A. (2001), 'Statement by USAID Administrator Andrew S. Natsios', Statement to the Third Least Developed Countries Conference, Brussels, 14 May.

Navarro V. (1998), 'Comment: Whose Globalization?' *American Journal of Public Health*, 88(5): 742.

Navarro V. (1999a), 'Health and Equity in the World in the Era of "Globalization"', *International Journal of Health Services*, 29(2): 215–26.

Navarro V. (1999b), 'Neoliberalism, "Globalization," Unemployment, Inequalities, and the Welfare State,' *International Journal of Health Services* 28(4): 607–82.

Nuffield Council on Bioethics (2002), *The ethics of research related to healthcare in developing countries*, London, May.

Nye J. (2002), *The Paradox of American Power: Why the World's Only Superpower Can't Go It Alone* (Oxford: Oxford University Press).

Ohmae K. (1990), *The Borderless World: Power and Strategy in the Interlinked Economy* (New York: HarperCollins).

Ohmae K. (1995), *The End of the Nation State, the Rise of Regional Economies* (New York: Free Press).

O'Neil C. (1996), 'Organic produce business skyrocketing, lots of room for growth', *CNN News*, 8 November. <www.cnn.com/HEALTH/indepth>

O'Neill J. (1990) 'AIDS as a Globalizing Panic' in Featherstone M. ed., *Global Culture* (London: Sage): 329–42

Ong E. and Glantz S. (2000), 'Tobacco Industry efforts subverting International Agency for Research on Cancer's second-hand smoke study,' *The Lancet*, 355, 8 April: 1253–9.

Oxfam (2000), 'Globalisation', Submission to the Government's White Paper on Globalisation, London, May.

PAHO (2001), 'Countries Need To Plan Effectively for "Deliberate Infections" – WHO Leader Urges Health Ministers', Press Release, Pan American Health Organization, 24 September.

Paton C. (1997), 'The Politics and Economics of Health Care Reform: Britain in Comparative Context' in Altenstetter C. and Bjorkman J. eds, *Health Policy Reform, National Variations and Globalization* (Basingstoke: Macmillan – now Palgrave Macmillan): 203–35.

Patterson K. (1996), *Pandemic Influenza 1700–1900, A Study in Historical Epidemiology* (Lanham, MD: Rowman & Littlefield)

Patz J., Epstein P., Burke T. and Balbus J. (1996), 'Global Climate Change and Emerging Infectious Diseases,' *Journal of the American Medical Association*, 275(3): 217–23.

Peters C. J. and Olshaker M. (1997), *Virus Hunter, Thirty Years of Battling Hot Viruses Around the World* (New York: Anchor Books).

Pfizer (2000), 'Pfizer Statement on Washington Post Clinical Trial Series', 17 December. <www.pfizer.com>

Pieterse J. (1995), 'Globalization as hybridization' in Featherstone M., Lash S. and Robertson R. eds, *Global Modernities* (London: Sage).

Pilling D. (1999a), 'Health returns to the Orient', *Financial Times*, 15 July: I–II.
Pilling D. (1999b), 'Locals beat back the big boys', *Financial Times*, 15 July: IV.
Pimentel D. (1986), 'Biological invasions of plants and animals in agriculture and forestry' in Mooney H. and Drake J. eds, *Ecology of Biological Invasions in North America and Hawaii* (New York: Springer-Verlag): 149–62.
Pimentel Simbulan N. (1999), 'The People's Health in the Era of Globalization', Paper presented to the Medical Action Group Forum on Human Rights, Manila, 6 December.
Pitt D. (1992), 'Power in the UN Bureaucracy: A New Byzantium', in Pitt D. and Weiss T. eds, *The Nature of UN Bureaucracies* (London: Croom Helm).
Polèse M. and Stren R. eds, (2000), *The Social Sustainability of Cities* (Toronto: University of Toronto Press/UNESCO).
Pollock A. and Price D. (2000), 'Rewriting the regulations: how the WTO could accelerate privatisation in health-care systems', *The Lancet*, 9 December, 356(9246): 1955–2000.
Popkin B. (1994), 'The Nutrition Transition in Low-Income Countries: An Emerging Crisis', *Nutrition Reviews*, 52(9): 285–98.
Porter J. and Ogden J. (1998), 'Social inequalities in the re-emergence of infectious disease' in Strickland S. and Shetty P. eds, *Human Biology and Social Inequality* (Cambridge: Cambridge University Press): 96–113.
Press E. and Washburn J. (2000), 'The Kept University', *Atlantic Monthly*, March.
Preston R. (1994), *The Hot Zone* (New York: Corgi Books).
Pretty J. (1994), 'Alternative systems of inquiry for a sustainable agriculture', *IDS Bulletin*, 25(2): 37–48.
Price-Smith A. (2002), *The Health of Nations: Infectious Diseases, Environmental Change, and Their Effects on National Security and Development* (Cambridge, Mass.: MIT Press).
Public Citizen (2000), *A Broken Record, How the FDA Legalized – and Continue to Legalize – Food Irradiation Without Testing for Safety*, Special Report, Public Citizen, The Cancer Prevention Coalition and Global Resource Action Center for the Environment, October. <http://www.citizen.org/publications> (accessed 29 March 2002)
Pyle G. F. (1986), *The Diffusion of Influenza, Patterns and Paradigms* (London: Rowman & Littlefield).
Radford T. (2002), 'World sickens as heat rises', *The Guardian*, 21 June.
RAND (2002), *Centre for Domestic and International Health Security* (Washington DC: RAND).
Rappole J. H., Deerrickson S. R. and Hubalek Z. (2000), 'Migratory birds and spread of West Nile virus in the Western Hemisphere', *Emerging Infectious Diseases*, 6(4): 319–28.
Raymond S. ed. (1997), *Global Public Health Collaboration: Organizing for a Time of Renewal* (New York: New York Academy of Sciences).
Reid S., Chalder T., Cleare A., Hotopf M. and Wessely S. (2000), 'Clinical review: Chronic fatigue syndrome', *British Medical Journal*, 320; 29 January: 292–6.
Reinicke W. (1997), 'Global Public Policy', *Foreign Affairs*, 76(6): 127–38.
Rhodes James R. (1994), *Henry Wellcome* (London: Hodder & Stoughton).
Roberts L. (1989), 'Disease and Death in the New World', *Science*, 8 December, 246 (4935): 1245–7.

Robertson R. (1992), *Globalization: Social Theory and Global Culture* (London: Sage).

Rockefeller Foundation/SIDA (2001), *Challenging Inequities in Health: From ethics to action* (Oxford: Oxford University Press).

Roddick A. (2001), Interview for 'Analysis: Globalising Doom', BBC Radio 4, 15 November.

Ruggie M. (1996), *Realignments in the Welfare State, Health Policy in the United States, Britain and Canada* (New York: Columbia University Press).

Rugman A. and Gestrin M. (1997), 'New Rules for Multilateral Investment', *International Executive*, 39(1): 21–33.

Ryan F. (1996), *Virus X, Understanding the Real Threat of the New Pandemic Plagues* (London: HarperCollins).

Sammels L. M., Lindsay M. D., Poidinger M., Coelen R. J. and Mackenzie J. S. (1999), 'Geographic distribution and evolution of Sindbis virus in Australia', *Journal of General Virology*, 80(3): 739–48.

Sassoon A. (1997), *Gramsci's Politics*, 2nd edition (Minneapolis: University of Minnesota).

Save the Children (1996), *Poor in Health* (London: SCF).

Schick A. (1998), 'Why most developing countries should not try New Zealand's reforms', *World Bank Research Observer*, 13(1): 123–31.

Schlosser E. (2002), *Fast Food Nation* (London: Penguin).

Scholte J. A. (1997a), 'Global capital and the state', *International Affairs*, July: 425–52.

Scholte J. A. (1997b) 'The Globalization of World Politics' in Baylis J. and Smith S. eds, *The Globalization of World Politics: An Introduction to International Relations* (Oxford: Oxford University Press): 13–30.

Scholte J. A. (2000), *Globalization, a Critical Introduction* (Basingstoke: Macmillan – now Palgrave Macmillan).

Schuftan C. (1999), 'Equity in health and economic globalisation', *Development in Practice*, 9(5): 610–14.

Schwartz P. and Gibb B. (1999), *When Good Companies Do Bad Things, Responsibility and Risk in an Age of Globalization* (New York: John Wiley).

Sen A. (2000), 'Freedom's market', *The Observer*, 25 June: 29.

Sen A. (2001), 'Slicing up the spoils', *The Guardian*, 19 July: 21.

Sen K. and Bonita R. (2000), 'Global health status: two steps forward, one step back', *Lancet*, 356, 12 August: 577–82.

Shakespeare W. (1591), *Romeo and Juliet.*

Shinn, E. A., Smith, G. W., Prospero, J. M., Betzer, P., Hayes, M. L., Garrison, V. and Barber R. T., (2000), 'African Dust and the Demise of Caribbean Coral Reefs', *Geophysical Research Letters*, 27(19): 3029–32.

Short C. (2001), 'Globalisation, Trade and Poverty Reduction in the Least Developed Countries', Speech by the UK Secretary of State for International Development at the Ministerial Roundtable on Trade and the Least Developed Countries, London, 19 March.

Shortridge K. F. (1999), 'The 1918 "Spanish" flu: pearls from swine?' *Nature Medicine*, April, 5(4): 384–5.

Shreeve J., *The Neanderthal Enigma, Solving the Mystery of Modern Human Origins* (New York: Viking, 1995).

SIDA (1997), *Sida Looks Forward – Sida's Programme for Global Development* (Stockholm: Swedish International Development Corporation Agency).

Singer P. and Benatar S. (2001), 'Beyond Helsinki: a vision for global health ethics', *British Medical Journal*, 322, 31 March: 747–8.

Singh K. (2002), 'War Profiteering, Anthrax, Drug Transnationals and TRIPS', Asia–Europe Dialogue Project <www.ased.org>

Smith R. P., Rand P. W., Lacombe E. H., Morris S. R., Holmes D. W. and Caporale D. A. (1996), 'Role of bird migration in the long-distance dispersal of *Ixodes dammini*, the vector of Lyme disease,' *Journal of Infectious Diseases*, 174(1): 221–4.

Smith A. (1776/1998), *An Inquiry into the Nature and Causes of the Wealth of Nations* (Oxford: Oxford Paperbacks).

Somasundaram M. (1996), 'Tobacco Companies in U.S. to Report Moderate-to-Strong First-Quarter Gains', *Wall Street Journal*, 9 April: A4.

Soros G. (2002), *On Globalization* (New York: PublicAffairs).

Spink W. (1978), *Infectious Diseases, Prevention and Treatment in the Nineteenth and Twentieth Centuries* (Dawson, Minn.: University of Minnesota Press).

Stephens J. (2000), 'As drug testing spreads, profits and lives hang in the balance', *Washington Post*, 17 December: A10.

Sterky G., Forss K. and Stenson B. (1996), *Tomorrow's global health organization: ideas and options* (Stockholm: Ministry of Foreign Affairs).

Stiglitz J. (1998), 'More Instruments and Broader Goals: Moving Towards the Post-Washington Consensus', *The 1998 WIDER Annual Lecture*, Helsinki, 7 January.

Stolberg S. (1998), 'Superbugs, the Bacteria Antibiotics Can't Kill', *New York Times Magazine*, 2 August: 42–7.

Strauss R. and Pollack H. (2001), 'Epidemic Increase in Childhood Overweight 1986–1998', *Journal of the American Medical Association*, 286(22), 12 December: 2845–8.

Tannahill R. (1973), *Food in History* (Harmondsworth: Penguin Books).

Tarlov A. (1996), 'Social determinants of health. The sociobiological translation', in Blane D., Brunner E. and Wilkinson R. eds, *Health and social organization. Towards a health policy for the twenty-first century* (London: Routledge): 71–93.

Tauran J. L. (2000), 'The Defence of Life in the Context of International Policies and Norms', Statement of Vatican, Rome, 11 February. <www.vatican.va/roman_curia...c_20000211_tauran-acdlife_en.html> (accessed 3 May 2001).

Taylor F. (1911), *The Principles of Scientific Management* (New York: Harper).

The Economist, '1897 and 1997, The century the earth stood still', *The Economist*, 18 December 1997.

Tong S., von Schirnding Y. and Prapamontol T. (2000), 'Environmental lead exposure: a public health problem of global dimensions', *Bulletin of the World Health Organization*, 78(9): 1068–77.

Torassa U. (2000), 'Finding HIV vaccine takes on new urgency: Little progress reported at AIDS conference', *San Francisco Examiner*, 13 July.

Tremolet S. (2001), 'Not a drop to spare', *The Guardian*, 26 September: 9 (Society).

Trounson A. (1997), 'Cloning: potential benefits for human medicine', *Medical Journal of Australia*, 167, 8 December: 568–69.

UK Department for International Development (2000), *Better Health for Poor People: Strategies for Achieving the International Development Targets* (London: HMSO).

UK Department of Health (2001), *The Health Effects of Climate Change* (London: Expert Group on Climate Change and Health).

UN Global Compact Office (2001), 'The Global Compact, Corporate Citizenship in the World Economy', <www.globalcompact.unorg>

UN Special Session on HIV/AIDS (2001), 'Global Crisis – Global Action, AIDS as a security issue', *Fact Sheet*, New York, 25–27 June.

UNAIDS (2001), *AIDS epidemic update December 2001* (Geneva: UNAIDS/WHO).

UNDP (1997), *Human Development Report 1997* (New York: UN Development Programme).

UNDP (1999), *Human Development Report 1999* (New York: UN Development Programme).

UNESCO (1998), *Declaration on Higher Education* (Paris: UN Educational, Scientific and Cultural Organization).

UNESCO (2000), *International Flows of Selected Cultural Goods 1980–98* (Paris: UNESCO Institute for Statistics).

UNFPA (1995), *World Urbanization Prospects: The 1994 Revision* (New York: UN Population Fund).

UNFPA (2002), *The State of the World's Population 2001* (New York: UN Population Fund).

UNHCR (2001), *Refugees by Numbers 2001* (Geneva: UN High Commissioner for Refugees). <www.unhcr.ch>

US Department of Agriculture (2000), 'Glickman announces national standards for organic foods', USDA News Release, Washington DC, 20 December. <http://www.ams.usda.gov/nop> (accessed 15 March 2002).

US Department of Energy (1992), *Primer on Molecular Genetics* (Washington DC: Human Genome Program).

US Department of Energy (1997), *Human Genome Program Report* (Washington DC: Office of Biological and Environmental Research).

US National Academy of Sciences (2001), *Abrupt Climate Change: Inevitable Surprises* (Washington DC: National Academy Press).

US National Intelligence Council (2000), *The Global Infectious Disease Threat and Its Implications for the United States* (Washington DC: National Intelligence Council).

US National Security Council (2000), 'International Health Affairs, Special Assistant to the National Security Advisor', <www.whitehouse.gov/nsc/>

USAID (1999), 'Women as Chattel: The Emerging Global Market in Trafficking', *Gender Matters Quarterly*, February. <www.usaid.gov/wid/pubs/q1.htm>

Van der Pijl K. (1989), 'Restructuring the Atlantic Ruling Class' in Gill S. ed., *Atlantic Relations: Beyond the Reagan Era* (Brighton: Wheatsheaf Books): 62–87.

Vaughan P., Mogedal S., Kruse S. E., Lee K., Walt G. and de Wilde K. (1995), *Cooperation for Health Development: Extrabudgetary funds in the World Health Organisation* (Oslo: Governments of Australia, Norway and the United Kingdom).

Vidal J. and Aglionby J. (2001), 'UN agency backs GM foods', *The Guardian*, 11 July: 12.

Violino B. (2001), 'E-Business Leaders Turn Web Efforts Into Profits', *InternetWeek.com*. <www.internetweek.com/100-01/intro.htm> (accessed 15 June 2002).

Vulliamy E. (2001), 'Empire hits back', *The Observer*, 15 July 2001: 23.

Wackernagel M. and Callejas A. (1995), 'The Ecological Footprints of 52 Nations (1995 data)', *Redefining Progress* <www.rprogress.org>

Wade R. (2001), 'Global inequality', *The Economist*, 28 April: 23–27.

Wagstaff A. and Watanabe N. (2000), *Socioeconomic Inequalities in Child Nutrition in the developing world* (Washington, DC: World Bank).

Walker S. (1997), 'Global Responses: The Search for Cures in the Development of Pharmaceuticals', *Indiana Journal of Global Legal Studies*, 5(1): 65–83.

Walker A. and Shipman P. (1996), *The Wisdom of Bones. In Search of Human Origins* (London: Weidenfeld & Nicolson).

Wallack L. and Montgomery K. (1992), 'Advertising for All by the Year 2000: Public Health Implications for Less Developed Countries', *Journal of Public Health Policy*, 13(2): 204–23.

Walters J. H. (1978), 'Influenza 1918: The Contemporary Perspective', *Bulletin of the New York Academy of Medicine*, October, 54(9): 855–64.

Ward K. and Lindheimer M. (1999), 'Genetic Factors in the Etiology of Preeclampsia/Eclampsia' in Lindheimer M., Roberts J. and Cunningham F. eds, *Chesley's Hypertensive Disorders in Pregnancy*, 2nd edition (New York: McGraw-Hill): 431–52.

Watkins K. (2002), 'Money talks', *The Guardian* [Society], 24 April: 10.

Watts S. (1997), *Epidemics and History, Disease, Power and Imperialism* (New Haven: Yale University Press).

Weick K. (1999), 'Sensemaking as an Organizational Dimension of Global Change' in Cooperider D. and Dutton J. eds, *Organizational Dimensions of Global Change, No Limits to Cooperation* (London: Sage): 39–56.

Weindling P. (1995), 'Introduction: constructing international health between the wars' in *International Health Organisations and Movements, 1918–1939* (Cambridge: Cambridge University Press): 1–16.

Weinstein L. (1976), 'Influenza – 1918, A Revisit?' *New England Journal of Medicine*, 6 May, 294(19): 1058–60.

Weisbrot M., Naiman R. and Kim J. (2001), 'The Emperor Has No Growth: Declining Economic Growth Rates in the Era of Globalization', *Briefing Paper*, Center for Economic Policy Research, Washington DC, May.

Weiss R. (1998), 'Babies in Limbo: Laws Outpaced by Fertility Advances', *Washington Post*, 8 February: A01.

Welch R. and Mitchell P. (2000), 'Food processing: a century of change', *British Medical Bulletin*, 56(1): 1–17.

Whitelegg J. (1993), 'Time Pollution', *Ecologist*, 23(4), July/August: 131–4.

WHO (1946), 'Constitution of the World Health Organization' in WHO (1994), *Basic Documents, Fortieth Edition* (Geneva): 1–18.

WHO (1958), *The First Ten Years of the World Health Organization* (Geneva: WHO).

WHO (1995), *WTO: What's in it for WHO?* (Geneva: WHO Task Force on Health Economics).

WHO (1996a), 'Noncommunicable Diseases, WHO Experts warn against inadequate prevention, particularly in developing countries', *Fact Sheet No. 106*, Geneva, March.

WHO (1996b), *World Health Report – Fighting Disease, Fostering Development* (Geneva: World Health Organization).

WHO (1997a), *Obesity, Preventing and Managing the Global Epidemic*, Technical Report Series (Geneva: WHO).

WHO (1997b), *Tobacco or Health, A Global Status Report* (Geneva: Tobacco Free Initiative).

WHO (1998a), 'Global infectious disease surveillance', *Fact Sheet No. 200*, Geneva, June. <www.who.int/inf-fs/fact200.html> (accessed 5 September 2000).

WHO (1998b), 'Health-for-all policy for the twenty-first century', Resolution WHA51.7, Fifty-First World Health Assembly, Geneva, 16 May.

WHO (1999a), '"Kobe Declaration" calls for a halt to the tobacco menace among women and children', *Press Release*, WHO/71, 18 November.

WHO (1999b) *Provisional list of participants*. First Meeting of the Working Group on the Framework Convention on Tobacco Control. A/FCTC/WG1/DIV/1.

WHO (1999c), *TB Advocacy, A Practical Guide* (Geneva: Global Tuberculosis Programme).

WHO (1999d), *World Health Report 1999: Making a Difference* (Geneva: World Health Organization).

WHO (2000a) *List of participants*. Intergovernmental Negotiating Body on the Framework Convention on Tobacco Control. Second session. A/FCTC/INB2/DIV/2 Rev.1.

WHO (2000b) *Participation of nongovernmental organizations in the Intergovernmental Negotiating Body*. Intergovernmental Negotiating Body on the Framework Convention on Tobacco Control. First session. A/FCTC/INB1/5 Para 4 and 6.

WHO (2000c), 'WHO, Internationally-Renowned Economists Launch Commission on Macroeconomics and Health', *Press Release*, 18 January.

WHO (2000d), 'WHO Issues New Healthy Life Expectancy Rankings', *Press Release*, 4 June.

WHO (2001a), *World Health Report 2001, Mental Health: New Understanding, New Hope* (Geneva: World Health Organization).

WHO (2001b), *The Tobacco Industry and Scientific Groups, ILSI: A Case Study* <www.who.int/geneva-hearings/inquiry.html>

WHO (2001c), 'WHO and Top Publishers announce Breakthrough on Developing Countries' access to leading biomedical journals', Press Release WHO/32, 9 July.

WHO Committee of Experts on Tobacco Industry Documents (2000), *Tobacco Industry Strategies to Undermine Tobacco Control Activities at the World Health Organization* (Geneva: Tobacco Free Initiative).

Wilding P. (1997), 'Globalization, Regionalism and Social Policy', *Social Policy and Administration*, 31(4): 410–28.

Wilkinson R. G. (1996), *Unhealthy Societies: The Afflictions of Inequality* (London: Routledge).

Williams A. (1999), 'Calculating the global burden of disease: time for a strategic reappraisal?' *Health Economics*, 8(1): 1–8

Williams F. (1998), 'Global advocate for health gets a shot in the arm', *Financial Times*, 19 May: 21.

Williamson J. ed. (1990), *Latin American Adjustment: How much has happened?* (Washington DC: Institute for International Economics).

Wilson M. (1995), 'Travel and the Emergence of Infectious Diseases', *Emerging Infectious Diseases*, 1(2): 39–46.

Wilson M., Levins R. and Spielman A. eds (1994), 'Disease in evolution: global changes and emergence of infectious diseases', *Annals of the New York Academy of Sciences*, 15 December, 740: 501–3.

Winston R. (2001), 'Why I weep for this baby – and the threat he poses to medicine', *Daily Mail*, 22 June: 12.

Wise J. (1997), 'Global food markets increase risk of infectious disease', *British Medical Journal*, 7 June, 314: 1641.

Wise R., Hart T., Cars O., Streulens M., Helmuth R., Huovinen P. and Sprenger M. (1998), 'Antimicrobial resistance is a major threat to public health', *British Medical Journal*, 317, 5 September: 609–10.

Wolf M. (2001), 'Growth makes the poor richer', *Financial Times*, 24 January: 25.

World Bank (1993), *World Development Report, Investing in Health* (Washington DC: International Bank for Reconstruction and Development).

World Bank (1998), *Poverty Reduction and the World Bank, Progress in Fiscal 1998* (Washington DC: International Bank for Reconstruction and Development).

World Bank (2000), 'Assessing Globalization', *World Bank Briefing Papers*, Washington DC, April.

World Bank (2001), *World Development Report, Attacking Poverty* (Washington DC: IBRD).

World Bank (2002), 'World Bank Intensifies Action Against HIV/AIDS', *Issue Briefs*, April. <www.worldbank.org/html/extdr/pb/pbaids.htm>

'World Bank is divided over poverty policy', *Nation* (Bangkok), 5 July 2000.

World Medical Association (1964), *Declaration of Helsinki* <www.ohsr.od.nih.gov/helsinki.php3>

World Tourism Organization (2001), Tourism Highlights 2001 (Madrid: WTO). <www.world-tourism.org/market_research/data/pdf/highlights updateengl.pdf>

WWF (2000), *Living Planet Report 2000* (London: Worldwide Fund for Nature).

WWF (2002), *Living Planet Report 2002* (London: Worldwide Fund for Nature).

Yach D. and Bettcher D. (1999), 'Globalization of Tobacco Marketing, Research and Industry Influence: Perspectives, trends and impacts on human welfare', *Development*, 42(4): 25–30.

Yach D. and Bettcher D. (2000), 'Globalisation of tobacco industry influence and new global responses', *Tobacco Control*, 9: 206–16.

Zarrilli S. and Kinnon C. eds. (1998), *International Trade in Health Services* (Geneva: WHO/UNCTAD).

Ziegler P. (1969), *The Black Death* (London: Alan Sutton).

Index

Lightning Source UK Ltd.
Milton Keynes UK
UKHW02f2310060318
319008UK00018B/435/P